Organic Acidurias

Previous Symposia of the Society for the Study of Inborn Errors of Metabolism.

1. Neurometabolic Disorders in Childhood. Ed. K. S. Holt and J. Milner 1963
2. Biochemical Approaches to Mental Handicap in Children. Ed. J. D. Allan and K. S. Holt 1964
3. Basic Concepts of Inborn Errors and Defects of Steroid Biosynthesis. Ed. K. S. Holt and D. N. Raine 1965
4. Some Recent Advances in Inborn Errors of Metabolism. Ed. K. S. Holt and V. P. Coffey 1966
5. Some Inherited Disorders of Brain and Muscle. Ed. J. D. Allan and D. N. Raine 1969
6. Enzymopenic Anaemias. Lysosomes and other papers. Ed. J. D. Allan, K. S. Holt, J. T. Ireland and R. J. Pollitt 1969
7. Errors of Phenylalanine Thyroxine and Testosterone Metabolism. Ed. W. Hamilton and F. P. Hudson 1970
8. Inherited Disorders of Sulphur Metabolism. Ed. Nina A. J. Carson and D. Noel Raine 1971

The Society exists to promote exchange of ideas between workers in different disciplines who are interested in any aspect of inborn metabolic disorders. Particulars of the Society can be obtained from the Editors of this Symposium.

Organic Acidurias

Proceedings of the Ninth Symposium of The Society for the Study of Inborn Errors of Metabolism

Edited by
J. STERN
and
C. TOOTHILL

CHURCHILL LIVINGSTONE
EDINBURGH and LONDON
1972

ISBN 0 443 00931 7

Any correspondence relating to this volume should be directed to the publishers at 15-17 Teviot Place, Edinburgh, EH1 2XX

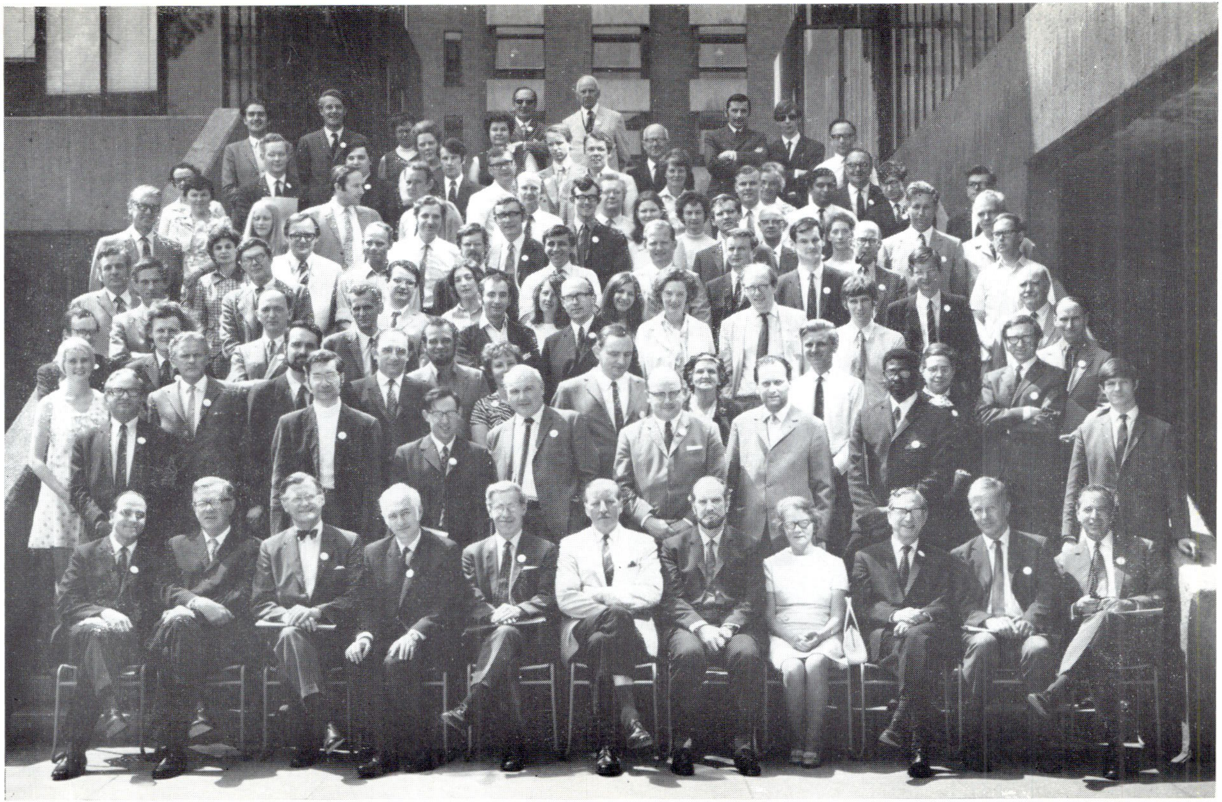

Delegates at the symposium. For key see numbered outline facing p. v and List of Participants with corresponding numbers in parentheses.

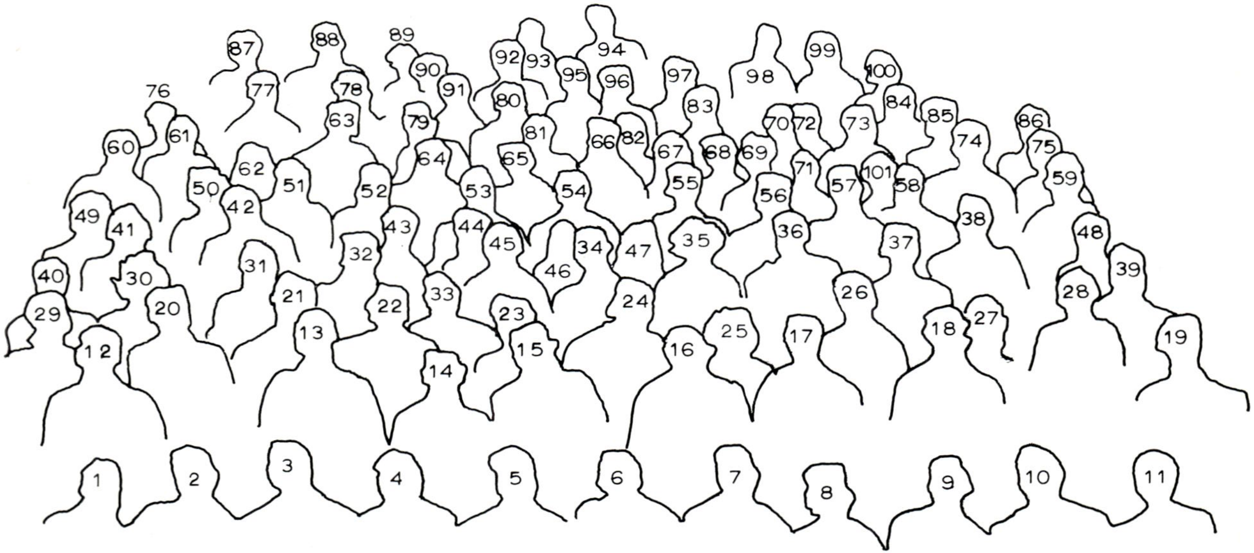

Key to Frontispiece

ACTIVE PARTICIPANTS IN SYMPOSIUM

Dr. J. D. ALLAN (6)
Department of Paediatrics, West Park Hospital, Macclesfield, England.

Dr. K. E. BAERLOCHER (63)
Universitäts-Kinderklinik, Kinderspital, 8032 Zurich, Switzerland.

Professor HELEN K. BERRY (92)
Department of Pediatrics, University of Cincinnati College of Medicine, Cincinnati, Ohio, U.S.A.

Professor H. BICKEL (11)
Universitäts-Kinderklinik, 6900 Heidelberg, Germany.

Dr. J. A. BLACK (81)
Children's Hospital, Western Bank, Sheffield S10 2TH, England.

Dr. D. P. BRENTON (85)
Department of Human Metabolism, University College Hospital, London, W.C.1, England.

Dr. D. BYRD (18)
Universitäts-Kinderklinik, 6900 Heidelberg, Germany.

Dr. NINA A. J. CARSON (83)
Department of Child Health, Grosvenor Road, Belfast BT12 6BJ, Northern Ireland.

Dr. H. C. CURTIUS (49)
Universitäts-Kinderklinik, Kinderspital, 8032 Zurich, Switzerland.

Dr. D. C. CUSWORTH (26)
Department of Human Metabolism, University College Hospital, London, W.C.1, England.

Dr. J. R. W. DYKES (87)
Department of Chemical Pathology, School of Medicine, Leeds LS2 9NL, England.

Professor L. ELDJARN (20)
Institute of Clinical Biochemistry, Rikshospitalet, Oslo, Norway.

Professor THEO GERRITSEN (60)
J. F. Kennedy Laboratory, University Wisconsin Medical Centre, Madison, Wisconsin 53706, U.S.A.

Dr. D. GOMPERTZ (14)
Department of Medicine, Royal Postgraduate Medical School, Ducane Road, London, W.12.

Dr. C. J. DE GROOT (69)
Department of Paediatrics, State University, 59 Oostersingel, Groningen, The Netherlands.

Dr. F. HANEFELD (56)
Children's Hospital of the Free University, 1 Berlin 19 (West), Germany.

Dr. F. HARRIS (100)
Department of Child Health, The Children's Hospital, Sheffield S10 2TH, England.

Dr. A. HODGKINSON
M.R.C. Mineral Metabolism Research Unit, Leeds General Infirmary, Leeds LS1 3EX, England.

Dr. K. S. HOLT (7)
The Wolfson Centre, Mecklenburgh Square, London, W.C.1, England.
Dr. EGIL JELLUM (52)
Institute of Clinical Biochemistry, Rikshospitalet, Oslo, Norway.
Professor J. H. P. JONXIS (2)
Department of Paediatrics, State University, 59 Oostersingel, Groningen, The Netherlands.
Dr. W. KOCHEN
Universitäts,Kinderklinik, 6900 Heidelberg, Germany.
Professor B. N. LA DU (42)
Department of Pharmacology, New York University Medical School, New York, 10016 NY, U.S.A.
Professor G. H. LATHE (5)
Department of Chemical Pathology, School of Medicine, Leeds LS2 9NL, England.
Dr. B. LEVIN (9)
Queen Elizabeth Hospital for Children, Hackney Road, London E2 8PS, England.
Dr. B. LINDBLAD (95)
Department of Clinical Chemistry, Sahlgren's Hospital, S-41345 Gothenburg, Sweden.
Professor SVEN LINDSTEDT (96)
Department of Clinical Chemistry, Sahlgren's Hospital, S-41345 Gothenburg, Sweden.
Dr. I. LOMBECK (23)
Children's Hospital, University of Dusseldorf, 4 Dusseldorf, Moorenstrasse, 5, Germany.
Dr. P. LUTZ (16)
Universitäts-Kinderklinik, 6900 Heidelberg, Germany.
Professor W. L. NYHAN (79)
Department of Pediatrics, University of California, La Jolla, California 92037, U.S.A.
Dr. C. A. PENNOCK (54)
Bristol Royal Infirmary, Bristol, England.
Professor THOMAS L. PERRY (10)
Department of Pharmacology, University of British Columbia, Vancouver 8, Canada.
Dr. R. J. POLLITT (30)
M.R.C. Unit for Metabolic Studies in Psychiatry, Middlewood Hospital, Sheffield S6 1TP, England.
Dr. D. N. RAINE (36)
Children's Hospital, Ladywood Middleway, Birmingham 16, England.
Dr. K. SCHÄRER (17)
Universitäts-Kinderklinik, 6900 Heidelberg 1, Germany.
Dr. J. W. T. SEAKINS (13)
Institute of Child Health, 30 Guilford Street, London WC1N 1EH, England.
Dr. L. SINCLAIR (22)
St. Stephen's Hospital, London, S.W.6, England.

Professor SELMA E. SNYDERMAN (50)
Department of Pediatrics, New York University Medical Center, School of Medicine, 550 First Avenue, New York, NY 10016, U.S.A.

Dr. J. SPENCER-PEET (88)
Department of Biochemistry, St. Bernard's Hospital, Southall, Middlesex.

Dr. J. STERN (4)
Queen Mary's Hospital for Children, Carshalton, England.

Dr. O. STOKKE (55)
Institute of Clinical Biochemistry, Rikshospitalet, Oslo, Norway.

Dr. C. TOOTHILL (1)
Department of Chemical Pathology, School of Medicine, Leeds LS2 9NL, England.

Dr. R. W. E. WATTS (3)
M.R.C. Clinical Research Centre, Watford Road, Harrow, Middlesex HA1 3UJ, England.

Also present on Frontispiece photograph:

Mrs. B. LEVIN, London (8); Dr. N. A. SYED, Walsall (12); Professor P.T. MOORE, Dublin (15); Mr. R. LOCKWOOD, Pontefract (19); Dr. R. TENCONI, Padua (21); Dr. G. BRUGMAN, Tubingen (24); Miss V. WILSON, Penistone (25); Dr. C. MARGOLES, London (27); Dr. V. DUBOWITZ, Sheffield (28); Miss A. DUCKWORTH, Leeds (29); Dr. S. P. M. VAN DER ZEE, Nijmegen (31); Dr. S. BEDONNEL, Nancy (32); Dr. C. BACCICHETTI, Padua (33); Dr. J. K. BROWN, Edinburgh (34); Dr. M. McMILLAN, London (35); Mr. B. FOWLER, Manchester (37); Dr. M. DURAN, Utrecht (38); Dr. D. E. NICHOLSON, Leeds (39); Dr. C. R. LEE, Sheffield (40); Dr. J. M. F. TRIJBELS, Nijmegen (41); Dr. VIDAILHET, Nancy (43); Dr. LEPOIRE, Nancy (44); Dr. HABEL Edinburgh (45); Miss M. GILES, Edinburgh (46); Mrs. J. TYFIELD, Bristol (47); Dr. T. WRIGHT, Sheffield (48); Dr. H. J. BREMER, Ulm (51); Dr. G. F. BATSTONE, Bristol (53); Dr. A. J. ROBBINS, Manchester (57); Dr. W. BLOM, Rotterdam (58); Dr. H. J. DAGENHARDT, Rotterdam (59); Miss M. MARTIN, Dublin (61); Miss V. FELL, Sheffield (62); Dr. J. B. HOLTON, Bristol (64); Dr. R. A. SAUNDERS, Cardiff (65); Mr. A. J. FRY, London (66); Miss J. R. COOKE, Birmingham (67); Dr. E. A. LAW, Aberdeen (68); Mr. J. G. JONES, Liverpool (70); Mr. B. HAWLEY, Sherbourne (71); Dr. M. B. MORRIS, Ulveston (72); Dr. I. B. SARDHARWALLA, Manchester (73); Dr. S. K. WADMAN, Utrecht (74); Dr. F. J. VAN SPRANG, Utrecht (75); Dr. V. P. COFFEY, Dublin (76); Dr. J. M. H. BUCKLER, Leeds (77); Dr. G. LINDSAY, Glasgow (78); Dr. G. LINDSTEDT, Gothenburg (80); Dr. G. DALE, Newcastle (82); Mr. J. T. IRELAND, Liverpool (84); Dr. J. H. RENWICK, London (86); Miss J. W. SUMMERSCALES, Leeds (89); Dr. M. S. McBEAN, Glasgow (90); Dr. I. SANDLE, Leeds (91); Mr. J. MILNER, Liverpool (93); Professor F. CHALLENGER, Leeds (94); Dr. R. M. TODD, Liverpool (97); Mr. MacCALLUM, Liverpool (98); Mr. P. MILNER, Liverpool (99); Dr. H. THOM, Aberdeen (101).

PREFACE

The warm reception accorded the Society's eighth symposium on sulphur metabolism amply vindicated the policy of henceforth confining the Annual Conference essentially to one theme. The topic chosen for the ninth symposium at Leeds was 'Organic Acidurias', a field in which the application of new techniques, particularly gas liquid chromatography and mass spectrometry, has led to the discovery of several new inborn errors of metabolism, some of which were presented at the symposium. Advances in technique have given a fresh impetus also to research into disorders of carbohydrate and amino acid metabolism where many of the metabolites involved are organic acids, and to studies in general of ninhydrin negative metabolites. Even the most sophisticated techniques can only detect cases if specimens are referred to the laboratory and part of the discussion centred on the clinical situations with a high index of suspicion which should prompt requests for appropriate investigations.

Once again we are very grateful to Mr. J. Milner of the Milner Scientific and Medical Research Company Liverpool for his generous support which made it possible to invite a number of eminent contributors from overseas. We also wish to thank the staff of the University of Leeds, academic and non-academic, for the warm welcome extended to participants in the symposium, and for much help with its organisation.

J. STERN
July, 1972 C. TOOTHILL

CONTENTS

KETOTIC HYPERGLYCINAEMIA

by

WILLIAM L. NYHAN, TOSHIYUKI ANDO, AND
KARSTEN RASMUSSEN

IT is clear that what we have called initially idiopathic hyperglycinaemia (Childs *et al.*, 1961), and then ketotic hyperglycinaemia (Nyhan *et al.*, 1967), is heterogeneous. A number of distinct diseases are now known that present with manifestations that would lead to a diagnosis of ketotic hyperglycinaemia. I believe that the extent of heterogeneity in this syndrome has just begun to be defined, and that a number of new diseases remain to be defined.

Clinical Considerations

Ketotic hyperglycinaemia may then be thought of as a generic or syndromic term. It is also of possible historical interest. We may, on the other hand, develop better ways of referring to the groups of patients involved. The clinical syndrome is one way to look at the problem. The cardinal features are shown in Fig. 1. The manifestations of non-ketotic hyperglycinaemia are shown for comparison. Patients with ketotic hyperglycinaemia develop repeated episodes of life threatening illness, characterised by ketosis and metabolic acidosis. Associated are vomiting and dehydration, and without vigorous treatment coma and death may ensue. The picture is much like that of diabetic acidosis, but without hyperglycaemia. Episodes may be precipitated by the intake of protein or by infection. Characteristically, onset is in early infancy, and we have felt that many patients may have died undiagnosed with what appeared to be overwhelming illness in the neonatal period. It is now clear that all patients do not develop mental retardation, and this does seem to be

Disorders presenting with hyperglycinemia

Clinical manifestations	
ketotic	*nonketotic*
Periodic ketoacidosis	Seizures
Neutropenia	Myoclonus
Thrombocytopenia	Hiccoughs
Osteoporosis	Respiratory acidosis
Developmental retardation	Failure to thrive
	Developmental retardation

FIG. 1. Cardinal clinical features of ketotic hyperglycinaemia and of nonketotic hyperglycinaemia.

related to careful management. It is also clear that all patients with this syndrome do not necessarily develop ketones in the urine in every acute episode of overwhelming illness. Obviously a number of conditions come immediately to mind which present with this clinical picture.

Glycine Concentrations in Blood

Another way of looking at the problem is to consider conditions in which there are elevated amounts of glycine in blood and urine. Obviously the two lists would not include all of the same conditions. Fig. 2 provides a list of conditions in which there is hyperglycinaemia. The condition we originally described as ketotic hyperglycinaemia is now generally recognised to be a primary propionic acidaemia. It is also widely known that patients with methylmalonic acidaemia have elevated concentrations of glycine in the blood. They do not always, but they do much of the time, and the elevations can be quite high. It is not so generally appreciated that patients with isovaleric acidaemia may not only have a clinical syndrome like that described above but may also have an elevated concentration of glycine in the blood. We have reported a patient with isovaleric acidaemia, recently published (Ando *et al.*, 1971a), who was initially referred to as a patient with ketotic hyperglycinaemia. It is our conviction that this list will grow.

Ketosis and metabolic acidosis
Ketotic hyperglycinaemia, propionic acidaemia—propionyl *CoA* carboxylase deficiency
Methylmalonic acidaemia
- B_{12} responsive
- B_{12} nonresponsive
- with homocystinuria

Isovaleric acidaemia
Nonketotic
Primary hyperglycinaemia
- Defective conversion of carbon 1 to CO_2 and carbon 2 to 1 carbon unit

FIG. 2. Classification of conditions which may present with hyperglycinaemia.

Amino Acid Intolerance

A listing of the components of protein which are capable individually of inducing symptoms of ketoacidosis in patients with ketotic hyperglycinaemia indicates that we are dealing with a multiple amino acid toxicity. Leucine, isoleucine, valine, threonine and methionine are all toxic, while the rest are innocuous. A similar list could be assembled in methylmalonic acidaemia except that leucine is non-toxic in this condition. Furthermore, we have now completed studies which indicate that isoleucine, valine, threonine and methionine are imperfectly metabolised in methylmalonic acidaemia and serve as sources of methylmalonic acid. This is consistent with what is known about the metabolism of the branched chain amino acids and methylmalonate.

The pattern of amino acid toxicity in ketotic hyperglycinaemia and the discovery of methylmalonic acidaemia led some to feel that ketotic hyperglycinaemia was methylmalonic acidaemia. However, analyses of body fluids in a number of patients revealed no methylmalonate. The likelihood that the pathway was involved suggested an evaluation of the metabolism of propionate.

Analysis of the Short Chain Organic Acids

Therefore, we and others undertook the exploration of the short chain organic acids in patients with ketotic hyperglycinaemia in the search for the presence or absence of abnormal concentrations of propionate. We studied patients with Dr George Donnell in Los Angeles and with Drs Nicholas Barnes, David Hull and Dennis Cottom in London. When I say 'we' I include my long time colleague, Dr Toshiyuki Ando, and, more recently, Dr Karsten Rasmussen. We have undertaken the development of methods for the systematic study of organic acids. These include the use of thin layer chromatography for screening and qualitative identification purposes, gas liquid chromatography, and an automatic organic acid analyser, which we had to build because these can no longer be purchased. Shortly, we expect to receive from the National Institutes of Health and Oak Ridge what is called a Body Fluid Analyser, an automatic instrument designed to separate large numbers of components of body fluids and to generate many unknown peaks. In the identification of these and other unknown compounds, we have been using an LKB instrument which combines gas liquid chromatography with the mass spectrometer. This instrument is enormously useful in the rapid and precise identification of organic compounds. Sample preparation is critical in the analysis of volatile acids in plasma.

Fig. 3 illustrates the gas liquid chromatography of the volatile acids of the plasma (Ando *et al.*, 1971b). V.B. and C.E. were patients with ketotic hyperglycinaemia and K.R. a control individual. The two top chromatograms are of the volatile acids of 0·2 ml whereas in the control we had to use four times that much. The numbered peaks were (1) solvent, (2) acetic acid, (3) propionic acid, (4) isobutyric acid, (5) butyric acid, and (6) isovaleric acid. A 6-foot Porapak Q-S glass U column was employed in a Packard 402 gas chromatograph. The striking difference between patient and control is in the marked elevation of peak 3, propionic acid. Isobutyric, butyric, and isovaleric acids were also present in the plasma in greater than normal concentration.

Propionic Acidaemia

The concentrations of propionate ranged from 10 to 24 μm/l, while in a

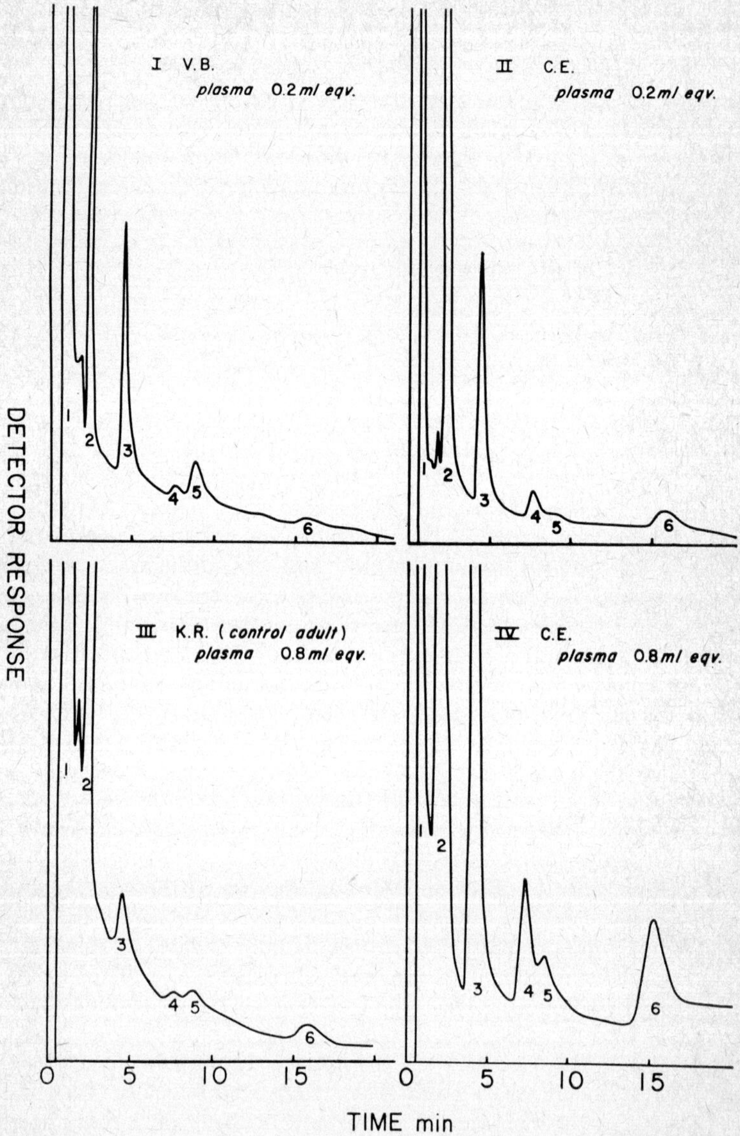

FIG. 3. Gas liquid chromatography of the organic acids of plasma. Patients V.B. and C.E. had ketotic hyperglycinaemia; K.R. was well. Peak 3 is that of propionic acid. Reprinted with permission from the *Journal of Pediatrics*.

series of controls the range was from 0·7 to 3·0, with a median of 1·2 μm/l. Thus concentrations in the patients were as much as twenty times the control level. Two patients studied with non-ketotic hyperglycinaemia had normal concentrations of propionate in the blood. Our patient with methylmalonic acidaemia had a concentration of 16 μm/l. It may be of interest to compare the concentrations of glycine in the plasma which ranged in three patients with ketotic hyperglycinaemia from 249 to 1150 μm/l, while the control mean was 146 μm/l. These studies of organic acidaemia establish the occurrence of propionic acidaemia as a characteristic of ketotic hyperglycinaemia. It is an even more reliable characteristic than the hyperglycinaemia, for one of our patients has had normal concentrations of glycine in the blood on a number of occasions. A syndrome of propionic acidaemia has been described by Hommes *et al.* (1968) in a patient who died at 5 days of age with severe metabolic acidosis but without hyperglycinaemia. We suspect that this was the same condition.

Propionate Oxidation

Defective metabolism of propionate can be demonstrated readily *in vivo* in these patients. We have carried out a study in which the patient was injected intravenously with Na propionate-1-^{14}C. Expired air was then collected at intervals over a two-hour period. Its CO_2 was trapped in ethanolamine in methylcellosolve and assayed for radioactivity and CO_2 content. In controls the specific activity of the CO_2 approximated 200,000 dpm/mM at the earliest time point. The curves then descended rapidly over the first 60 minutes. In contrast in a patient with ketotic hyperglycinaemia the curve was relatively flat, rising very slowly throughout the 2 hours, as if something was being slowly synthesised that then served as a source of CO_2. The curve for the patient with methylmalonic acidaemia was intermediate, certainly lower than normal but much higher than the patient with ketotic hyperglycinaemia, and the curve was of relatively normal configuration.

Oxidation of Glycine

These observations clearly indicate a defect in propionate metabolism that is consistent with the propionic acidaemia. It is also possible to demonstrate in the same way a defect in glycine metabolism that is consistent with the hyperglycinaemia. We have carried out a number of studies of glycine metabolism *in vivo* (Ando *et al.*, 1968). In control individuals glycine-1-^{14}C is rapidly converted to CO_2 *in vivo*. The presence of a large glycine pool, as produced by constant infusion of non-isotopic glycine, would be expected to dilute the isotope, but it also increases the rate of oxidation, and the specific activities are higher. We have previously reported that in non-ketotic hyperglycinaemia there is a defect in the conversion of the first carbon of glycine to CO_2. Two of the patients with ketotic hyperglycinaemia whom we have studied were found to convert glycine-l-^{14}C to CO_2 at about the rate observed in non-ketotic hyperglycinaemia. In the third, the defect was much less prominent except at the earliest time point after which the specific activity rose, so that by 60 minutes the values in this patient could not be distinguished from controls. These data speak for heterogeneity in this condition.

It is not possible to describe the defect in glycine metabolism more fully or to assess whether or not it is primary. It could be that the defect in glycine metabolism is secondary to that in propionate metabolism. It could be the other way around. It could also be that both are secondary, possibly to a defect in co-factor synthesis.

Propionate Metabolism *in vitro*

Defective oxidation of propionate can also be demonstrated *in vitro*. Hsia *et al*. (1969) has reported this in leukocytes. We have studied it in fibroblasts. We incubated intact fibroblasts in bicarbonate buffer with Na propionate-l-^{14}C for 90 minutes at 37°C. The values found in the patient for isotope in CO_2 approximated one-tenth those of controls. Cells of a patient with non-ketotic hyperglycinaemia carried out this conversion normally.

These observations suggested a defect in the enzyme propionyl CoA carboxylase. We have assayed the activity of this enzyme in extracts of fibroblasts grown in cell culture. In the patient we studied there was virtually no activity. Similarly, no activity was reported by Hsia *et al.* (1970) in extracts of fibroblasts from a patient with ketotic hyperglycinaemia and very low activity was reported by Gompertz *et al.* (1970) in a mitochondrial preparation from the liver of a patient. These observations provide a site for a molecular understanding of this disease. The site could, of course, be other than the propionyl CoA carboxylase apoenzyme, as well as in the primary structure of this protein. It is also possible that the sites differ in different patients.

Metabolic Products of Propionate *in vivo*

Information on the metabolic patterns of these patients is beginning to accumulate from the study of the urine collected during the tracer studies discussed above. In one such study, following the administration of labelled propionate to a patient with ketotic hyperglycinaemia a new spot was found next to citrate on a paper chromatogram of the organic acids of the urine. The urine was acidified and subjected to continuous extraction into ether, followed by concentration and chromatography on Whatman No. 1 paper in two dimensions (ethanol, NH_3, H_2O, and propanol, formic acid). The spot was found to be radioactive by radioautography.

The urine was then studied on the organic acid analyser. Two peaks were found which were highly labelled, before malate and after cis-aconitate. The most highly radioactive peak was greater in activity than any of the other peaks in the urine, including propionate, after the administration of labelled propionate. The fractions were isolated and analysed on the gas chromatography-mass spectrometer. The mass spectrum fits a molecular size of citric acid plus 14. This would suggest that there is a methyl group in addition to the citrate molecule. The data would fit a structure we could call methyl citrate (Fig. 4) or homocitrate. Methyl citrate might be considered an analogous molecule to methylmalonic acid. Homocitrate would be the expected product if acetyl CoA underwent a condensation with α-ketoglutarate that was analogous to its condensation with oxalacetate. If, on the other hand, propionyl CoA condensed with oxalacetate, the expected product would be methyl citrate. In either case we would need a new condensing enzyme. The familiar one is highly specific for both oxalacetate and acetyl CoA.

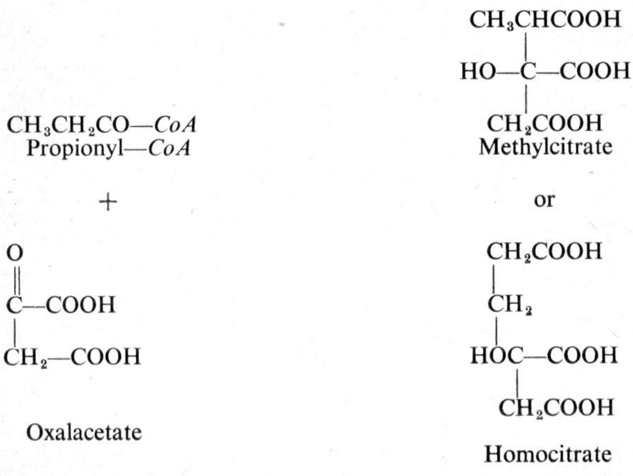

FIG. 4. Postulated pathway which could lead to the synthesis of methyl citrate or homocitrate.

Another major peak of radioactivity was found at 180 minutes in both ketotic hyperglycinaemia and in methylmalonic acidaemia. There was no radioactivity in this area in the control. The radioactivity corresponded to a peak of acid that was identified as pyrrolidone carboxylic acid, or pyroglutamic acid. However, when the fractions involved were chromatographed on paper the pyrrolidone carboxylic acid and the radioactivity were readily separated. The trimethylsilyl derivatives were made and subjected to gas chromatography, which revealed the peak of pyrrolidone carboxylic acid and a new, fast moving peak. The mass spectrum was consistent with a structure of 3-hydroxypropionate.

Summary

We have considered ketotic hyperglycinaemia as a syndrome of overwhelming illness, presenting very early in life. The clinical syndrome can be caused by a number of diseases not all of which have hyperglycinaemia, at least not all of the time. We feel that the extent of heterogeneity has just begun to be defined. A narrower view of the disorder is provided by the documentation of propionic acidaemia as a uniform chemical characteristic. Therefore, what we originally described as ketotic hyperglycinaemia should more properly be termed propionic acidaemia, or propionic acidaemia with hyperglycinaemia, or hyperglycinaemia with propionic acidaemia. In this condition there is defective oxidation of glycine and propionate *in vivo*. Defective oxidation of propionate has been demonstrated *in vitro*, and there is a defect in the enzyme propionyl CoA carboxylase. A compound was found in the urine which was formed from propionate and which had a structure consistent with methyl citrate. This compound was especially prominent in ketotic hyperglycinaemia but was also found in methylmalonic acidaemia. In both conditions 3-hydroxypropionate was found as a product of propionate, which was also absent in control individuals.

REFERENCES

Ando, T., Klingberg, W. G., Ward, A. M., Rasmussen, K. & Nyhan, W. L. *Pediat. Res.* (1971a), **5**, 478.

Ando, T., Nyhan, W. L., Gerritsen, T., Gong, L., Heiner, D. C. & Bray, P. F. (1968) *Pediat. Res.*, **2**, 254.

Ando, T., Rasmussen, K., Nyhan, W. L., Donnell, G. & Barnes, N. D. (1971b) *J. Pediat.*, **78**, 827.

Childs, B., Nyhan, W. L., Borden, M. A., Bard, L. & Cooke, R. E. (1961) *Pediatrics*, **27**, 670.

Gompertz, D., Storrs, C. N., Bau, D. C. K., Peters, T. J. & Hughes, E. A. (1970) *Lancet*, **1**, 1140.

Hommes, F. A., Kuipers, J. R. G., Elema, J. D., Jansen, J. F. & Jonxis, J. H. P. (1968) *Pediat. Res.*, **2**, 519.

Hsia, Y. E., Scully, K. J. & Rosenberg, L. E. (1969) *Lancet*, **1**, 757.

Hsia, Y. E., Scully, K. J. & Rosenberg, L. E. (1970) *Proc. Soc. pediat. Res.*, **40**, 26.

Nyhan, W. L., Ando, T. & Gerritsen, T. (1967). In Nyhan, W. L. (ed.), *Amino Acid Metabolism and Genetic Variation*, p. 97. New York: McGraw-Hill Book Co.

METHYLMALONIC ACIDURIA METHYLMALONYL CoA MUTASE ACTIVITY IN LEUCOCYTES

by

B. LEVIN, V. G. OBERHOLZER, AND E. ANN BURGESS

METHYLMALONIC aciduria was first described by Oberholzer *et al.*, in 1967, and the clinical features of this disease are well exemplified by the first two cases. Both had, from the first weeks of life, intermittent vomiting which was at first fairly frequent, but later, with treatment, was less so. Both had an associated metabolic acidosis. Initially these episodes of vomiting and acidosis were considered to be due to infection with which they tended to be associated. It was later realised that infection, if present, was only slight, and was sometimes absent. In both hepatomegaly was present. In one child, a boy, physical and mental retardation was obvious by the time he died when 2 years old. The second child, a girl, was considered to be retarded physically and mentally at 4 months of age, but re-assessment at 2 and 4 years of age showed that she had regained a normal state probably because of the close supervision and treatment she had received.

The most striking presenting feature is the persistent metabolic acidosis. In both children this was at first thought to be a renal tubular acidosis and was treated as such. During severe episodes, the CO_2 content of the plasma could fall as low as 6 meq/l but was usually about 12 meq/l without treatment. Ketosis was always present. The level of total ketone bodies in the plasma was usually raised under fasting conditions and in periods of acute illness was markedly so. The hydrogen ion clearance index in one child measured on three occasions between 6½ and 17 months of age was very low, between 0·26 and 0·59, compared with a normal value of 1·2 or more. A similar test was not performed on the other child, but it was thought since the urine pH could be as low as 4·8 when there was a very severe acidosis, that the renal ability to excrete H^+ was not reduced. In both children, both the urea and creatinine clearances were severely impaired, but in the child that survived these had greatly improved by 6 years of age.

The cause of the chronic renal disease is not certain. There is some slight evidence that methylmalonic acid may be toxic to the kidney (Corley & Rose, 1926), but it is more likely that the impaired metabolism of this acid in the kidney with its consequent effect on the citric acid cycle, results in renal dysfunction. Uric acid excretion is inhibited by many organic acids, e.g. lactic acid, and the high plasma uric acid level ranging between 8·0 and 23·6 mg per 100 ml found on various occasions in our case, may be due to a similar inhibition by methylmalonic acid.

The level of methylmalonic acid in the fasting plasma can be very high, up to 27·5 mg per 100 ml, and the excretion is very great, up to 6 g per day, even on a restricted protein intake. The level in cerebro-spinal fluid was also high, about the same as in the plasma. Propionic acid excretion was also raised, to 87·0 and 95·0 mg per day measured on two occasions, i.e. well over 100 times the normal. The acetic acid excretion was within normal limits.

Metabolic Block

The transformations from propionyl CoA to succinyl CoA are shown in Fig. 1. D-methylmalonyl CoA arising from the carboxylation of propionyl CoA is transformed by a racemase to its L-enantiomorph, which is then converted to succinyl CoA by methylmalonyl CoA mutase in the presence of its co-enzyme, 5′-deoxyadenosylcobalamin. The accumulation of very high amounts of methylmalonic acid in plasma and cerebrospinal fluid indicates the block to be in the transformation of the CoA derivative, to succinyl CoA. The possible causes for this defective transformation were first clearly stated in the original publication (Levin *et al.*, 1966; Oberholzer *et al.*, 1967). They were (*a*) a defective racemase, (*b*) a defective mutase, (*c*) a lack of the specific cobamide required for the final step, the conversion of L-methylmalonyl CoA to succinyl CoA.

There was some evidence against the third possibility. (*a*) The blood and cerebrospinal fluid levels of methylmalonic acid were very high; (*b*) the plasma level of vitamin B_{12} was actually higher than normal; and (*c*) the amount of methylmalonic acid excreted in 24 hours far exceeded the amount excreted in vitamin B_{12} deficiency. Furthermore, in one of our cases an intramuscular injection of 2 mg vitamin B_{12} caused little or no change in the amount of methylmalonic acid excreted. In 24 hours prior to the injection, 4·8 g methylmalonic acid were excreted; yet in the 24 hours immediately following the injection, 4·0 g were excreted. Little effect was discernible even when the 3-hourly excretion rate following the injection was determined. A further period of 1 mg per day injections of vitamin B_{12} for 4 days resulted in a relatively small decrease from 7·0 g/day to 5·85 g in methylmalonic acid excretion. Finally, the enzyme activity was not increased by the addition of cyancobalamin to the assay mix. However, some examples of this condition have been discovered, which do respond to vitamin B_{12} injections by a marked reduction in methylmalonic acid excretion (Rosenberg *et al.*, 1968).

Overall Conversion of Propionyl CoA in Leucocytes

This has been followed by incubating propionyl CoA with leucocyte suspension and $Na_2{}^{14}CO_3$ for 20 minutes. The extracted acids were

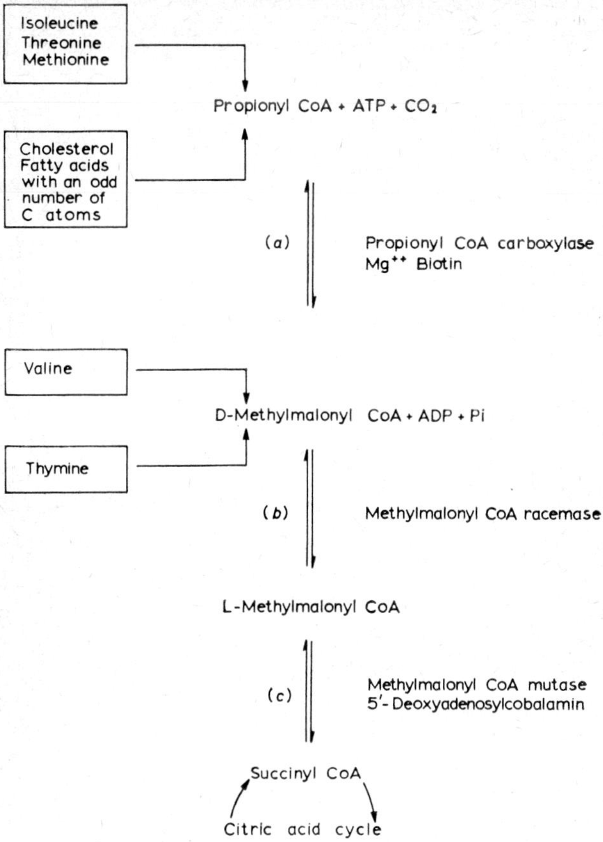

FIG. 1. Metabolism of propionic acid

separated by high voltage paper electrophoresis, the relevant sections cut, and the radioactivity counted. The results on the leucocytes from two affected children, from the parents of one of them, and from five normal adults are shown in Table I. In all cases, methylmalonyl CoA was formed, but the amount of methylmalonic acid remaining at the end of incubation was higher in both affected children, as well as in the parents of one of them, suggesting a defective metabolism of methylmalonic acid. Although the amount of methylmalonic acid formed varied in three separate experiments, all demonstrated an inability to convert methylmalonic acid to succinyl CoA.

Assay of Methylmalonyl CoA Mutase Activity in Leucocytes

In order to elucidate the site of the metabolic block as well as to

Table I. *Overall metabolism of propionyl CoA in leucocytes*

Subject	*Methyl* ^{14}*C malonate cpm/10*^{8}*cells/20 min.*	^{14}*C-Labelled S+F+M cpm/10*^{8}*cells/20 min.*
S.H.	8050	778
S.H. + Vit. B_{12}	8410	587
D.D.	4750	722
Mother of S.H.	8050	1100
Father of S.H.	2380	870
Controls 1	330	137
2	778	260
3	1440	352
4	1239	603
5	1139	444

The incubation mixture contained 50 mM Tris buffer, pH 7·4; 3 mM $MgCl_2$, 3 mM ATP, 5 mM reduced glutathione, 1mM propionyl CoA, 10 mM $Na_2C^{14}O_3$ (2μCi) and approximately 21×10^6 white cells, homogenised in a small volume of 40 mM Tris buffer, pH 8·0 containing 1 mM reduced glutathione. The total volume was 1 ml.
S = succinate; F = fumarate; M = malate

attempt to assay the mutase activity a direct measurement of the conversion of methyl[^{14}C]malonyl CoA into succinyl CoA in leucocytes was made, using a racemic mixture of D- and L-methylmalonyl CoA. This would differentiate between a defective racemase (reaction *b*) and a defective mutase (reaction *c*). If both enzymes are normal, the conversion of both D and L forms will be complete; if the racemase alone is defective, only half the added substrate can react. Finally, if the mutase is defective, no reaction will occur. The method of Cannata *et al.* (1965) for the assay of the activity of liver methylmalonyl CoA mutase was applied to leucocyte homogenates. Methyl[^{14}C]malonyl CoA was prepared by incubating a mixture of propionyl CoA, $Na_2{}^{14}CO_3$ and propionyl CoA carboxylase, prepared from ox liver, in Tris/HCl buffer containing $MgCl_2$, KCl, ATP, phosphoenolpyruvate and pyruvate kinase. It was converted to the racemic mixture by heating at 100° for 25 minutes. The leucocyte suspension was incubated with a preparation containing approximately 250 mμmoles of methyl[^{14}C]malonyl CoA in tris/HCl buffer. Aliquots were withdrawn at intervals of 2½ minutes, with a final one at 20 minutes. The amounts of methylmalonic and succinic acids in each of these aliquots were determined by high voltage electrophoretic separation on paper in pyridine acetic acid buffer pH 3·5 and counting the radioactivity in the relevant spots. The results obtained in two cases of methylmalonic aciduria, the parents of one affected child, and in five normal adults are shown (Table II and Fig. 2). Essentially no enzyme activity was detected in both affected children. In both the parents of one of the children, the methylmalonyl CoA mutase activity was below the lower limit of normal, suggesting the heterozygote state.

Table II. *Methylmalonyl CoA mutase activity in leucocytes*

	Units
S.H.	0
D.D.	0
Mother of S.H.	15·4
Father of S.H.	5·2
Normal Adults	63·0, 18·8, 92·8, 36·6, 54·0
Mean	53·04

1 unit = 1 mμmole methylmalonic acid utilised/min./10^8cells

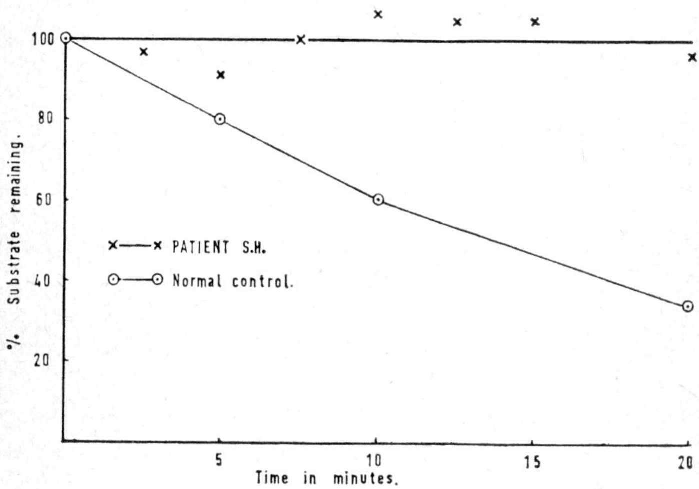

FIG. 2. The mixture containing 0·3 ml of a leucocyte suspension, 1·5 ml of a preparation with approximately 250 mμmoles methylmalonyl CoA prepared from propionyl CoA and $Na_2{}^{14}CO_3$, and 1·2 ml 0·25 M tris/HC1 pH 7·5 was incubated for 30 min. at 37°.

Effect of Vitamin B_{12} on Methylmalonyl CoA Mutase Activity

Although methylmalonyl CoA mutase activity in the leucocyte homogenate from the affected child was not increased in the presence of added cyancobalamin, this might have been due to the fact that 5′-deoxyadenosylcobalamin, the specific co-enzyme in the reaction, had not been formed from the inactive cyancobalamin. The assay was therefore repeated, with the separate addition of both 5′-deoxyadenosylcobalamin and methylcobalamin, the incubation being carried out in subdued light to avoid any breakdown of the specific co-enzyme. The results are shown in Table III. No mutase activity was observed when no co-factor was added or when methylcobalamin was present but a significant activity, 9·5 mμmoles/10^8 cells/min., was induced in the presence of 5′-deoxyadenosylcobalamin in a concentration of 10^{-5} M. This is approximately the same activity as that found in the parents of the affected child, but is very much less than in normal controls. Since injection of large doses of cyancobalamin failed to reduce methylmalonic acid excretion in this patient, she cannot be considered to be a B_{12} dependent type. The induction of mutase activity in the leucocyte homogenate is presumably due to the high concentration of added 5′-deoxyadenosylcobalamin. The results therefore indicate that, in leucocytes at least, an increased mutase activity in the presence of high levels of co-enzyme does not necessarily prove vitamin B_{12} dependency. Morrow *et al.* (1969) also demonstrated an increased metabolism of methylmalonic acid in the presence of added co-enzyme by liver homogenates from children presumed to have the unresponsive variant of methylmalonic aciduria, although the increase was much greater with the presumed B_{12} dependent variant.

Table III. *Methylmalonyl CoA mutase activity in leucocytes: effect of addition of 5′-deoxyadenosylcobalamin and methylcobalamin*

Patient	*Addition*	*Activity (mμmoles/10⁸cells/min.)*
S.H.	Nil	0
	Methylcobalamin	0
	5′-deoxyadenosylcobalamin	9·5

Rosenberg *et al.* (1969) found that cultured skin fibroblasts from two patients suffering from the B_{12} dependent condition failed to convert methylmalonyl CoA to succinyl CoA and contained only about 10 per cent of the mean amount of 5′-deoxyadenosylcobalamin of normal controls. Morrow *et al.* (1969) found the cobamide content of the liver of one out of four patients with methylmalonic aciduria who died to be extremely low, the others having apparently normal amounts. It has therefore been suggested (Rosenberg *et al.*, 1969) that there is a defect of synthesis or metabolism of the vitamin in the B_{12} dependent form.

If this is so, it seems surprising that the amount of methylmalonic acid excreted is so much greater than in vitamin B_{12} deficiency. Such a result, however, would be explicable if there were different defects in the apo-enzyme in both variant types. This would imply the existence of two different mutations affecting the apo-enzyme, one involving the binding site of the substrate, and the other that of the co-enzyme. The decreased co-enzyme content of liver or cultured skin fibroblasts in the Vitamin B_{12} responsive type could be explained by the inability of the defective apo-enzyme to bind the co-enzyme. The specific biochemical basis for the vitamin B_{12} responsive variant has not therefore been settled.

Excretion of Methylmalonic Acid in Normals and in Parents of Affected Child

The method used for the assay of the small amounts of methylmalonic acid in normal urine was in principle as follows. An aliquot of the 24-hours specimen of urine is made alkaline, concentrated *in vacuo* to one-tenth its volume, acidified and then extracted three times with ether. The methylmalonic acid is re-extracted from the ether solution by shaking with 5 N ammonia, and a small aliquot of this extract is chromatographed on paper, using ethanol-ammonia-water as solvent system. The zone of paper corresponding to methylmalonic acid is eluted with very dilute NaOH and the methylmalonic acid is determined colorimetrically by a modification of the method of Oberholzer *et al.* (1967). The method is very sensitive and gives excellent recovery.

The results in normal infants and children as well as in adults are shown in Table IV, together with the methylmalonic acid excretion in both parents of an affected child. Not surprisingly, the amount excreted varies with age, being lower, the younger the age, and highest with adults. These levels are well below the upper limit of those reported in the literature. The excretion of methylmalonic acid by both parents is in excess of the upper limit of the normal which would suggest that this measurement can be used to detect the heterozygote state.

Table IV. *Methylmalonic acid excretion*

Normal children and adults

Age	*No. of subjects*	*MMA mg/day*	*Range mg/day*
Up to 1 year	6	0·4	0·20–0·84
1 to 5 years	4	0·96	0·65–1·2
5 to 14 years	7	1·7	0·7 –3·1
Adults	7	2·8	2·3 –3·6

Parents of Affected Child

	MMA mg/day	*Before 10g Valine mg MMA/day*	*After 10g Valine mg MMA/day*
Mother	9·0, 6·3	6·8	7·2
Father	5·4	4·7	4·6

An earlier attempt to stress in the parents the metabolic pathway involved by a loading dose of sodium propionate yielded an inconclusive result partly because it induced vomiting, and also because at that time no satisfactory method for the assay of low levels of methylmalonic acid in urine had been devised. However, a later test showed no increase in the amount of methylmalonic acid excreted in the 24 hours following a loading dose of 10 g valine.

REFERENCES

Cannata, J. J. B., Focesi, A. Jr., Mazumder, R., Warner, R. C. & Ochoa, S. (1965) *J. biol. Chem.*, **240**, 3249.

Corley, R. C. & Rose, W. C. (1926) *J. Pharmacol. exp. Ther.*, **27**, 165.

Levin, B., Oberholzer, V. G., Burgess, E. Ann & Young, Winifred, F. (1966) *Lancet*, **2**, 1415.

Morrow, G. III, Barness, L. A., Cardinale, G. J., Abeles, R. H. & Flaks, J. G. (1969) *Proc. Nat. Acad. Sci.* (*Wash.*), **63**, 191.

Oberholzer, V. G., Levin, B., Burgess, E. Ann & Young, Winifred F. (1967) *Arch. Dis. Childh.*, **42**, 492.

Rosenberg, L. E., Lilljeqvist, A. C. & Hsia, Y. E. (1968) *New Engl. J. Med.*, **278**, 1319.

Rosenberg, L. E., Lilljeqvist, A. C. & Hsia, Y. E. (1968) *Science*, **162**, 805.

DISCUSSION
(of Papers by Professor Nyhan and Dr Levin)

de Groot (*Groningen*). The Dutch patient with propionic acidaemia referred to by Professor Nyhan did not have a raised blood glycine level on his second day of life, in contrast to most patients with the ketotic form of hyperglycinaemia. Apart from this he is like other patients with ketotic hyperglycinaemia.

Professor Nyhan, you indicated that one of your patients with propionic acidaemia also had a defect in glycine oxidation. Do you suggest that this is another basic disorder or a secondary defect? The connection between propionyl CoA carboxylase and glycine metabolism is not immediately apparent.

Nyhan (*La Jolla*). I suspect that the defect in glycine oxidation is secondary. I also have a problem seeing the connection, but it is of fundamental importance to discover why a patient with a defect in propionylCoA carboxylase might have a secondary elevation of glycine concentrations in body fluids or a secondary defect in glycine oxidation.

I think the key to this understanding is the patient with methylmalonic acidaemia who clearly does not have a primary defect in glycine metabolism but who does have hyperglycinaemia. Patients with isovaleric acidaemia can do this same kind of thing. These phenomena must be telling us something, but they do not yet seem to be telling us what the answer is. The implication, in my view, is that the defect in glycine oxidation is almost certainly a secondary defect in the patient with ketotic hyperglycinaemia. Relevant to that, may I expand a little on glycine metabolism. In our studies on glycine metabolism in nonketotic hyperglycinaemia, the oxidation of the first carbon of glycine to CO_2 was about the same as that we found in ketotic hyperglycinaemia. The key finding in nonketotic hyperglycinaemia came from the studies on the metabolism of the second carbon atom of glycine which is normally converted quite rapidly to the third carbon atom of serine, indicating that it must go through a one carbon tetrahydrofolate intermediate. In the patient with nonketotic hyperglycinaemia that conversion of the second carbon atom of glycine to the third carbon atom of serine is not made. Now, to come back to the patient with ketotic hyperglycinaemia, the metabolism of the second carbon atom of glycine to the third carbon atom of serine is perfectly normal. Metabolically, these are two quite different conditions.

Eldjarn (*Oslo*). In Professor Nyhan's presentation hydroxypropionic acid and methyl citrate figure prominently. Have you done any experiments to ensure that hydroxypropionic acid is not an artefact? In our systems hydroxypropionic acid is produced from traces of water, methanol, hydrochloric acid and diazomethane.

The formation of homocitrate reminds me of the work of Sir Rudolph Peters (*Biochemical Lesions and Lethal Synthesis*, 1963, Oxford, Pergamon) on fluoroacetate poisoning via the formation of fluorocitrate. Could it be that homocitrate similarly interferes with the citric acid cycle and that some of the symptoms could be explained in this way?

Nyhan (*La Jolla*). Thank you very much for your comment and for reminding me about fluoroacetate and its condensation. One of the earliest things I worked with in the laboratory was fluoroacetate, and I learned a considerable respect for it. As you know, it is extremely toxic. It has been used in Africa as a rat poison; it is, as documented by Peters, condensed to fluorocitrate and acts as inhibitor of the citric acid cycle. We have told you this morning the sum total of our information up to a week or so ago, so that the experiment you suggest has not been carried out. However, it certainly will be.

We have been puzzled, from the time we saw the first patient with the ketotic hyperglycinaemia syndrome, with the mechanism of ketosis in these children. I think that whether you look at methylcitrate or homocitrate, if you will, as a way of draining of four carbon acids and thus depleting the citric acid cycle of the material with which to condense acetylCoA, or whether you look at it as a toxic compound like fluorocitrate, it would provide a good way of explaining the ketosis which is central to all these conditions. This is a very exciting aspect of this new observation.

Gerritsen (*Madison*). In the infant at risk from hyperglycinaemia it is the glycine/alanine ratio in the plasma which must be watched. This is less than 1 in normal infants. In the early stages of ketotic hyperglycinaemia the serum glycine level may be barely increased but the glycine/alanine ratio is greater than 1.

Nyhan. I certainly would second that comment. We have had experience with at least two patients in whom we have found normal glycine levels on more than one occasion and for relatively prolonged periods of time.

This was particularly exemplified by George Donnell's case in which they knew that the patient was a sibling of a known patient with ketotic hyperglycinaemia who had died of the disease. It was approximately six weeks before that patient developed consistent elevations of the serum glycine.

This is, of course, further evidence of the fact that the glycine abnormality is probably secondary. It also points out the difficulty of making a diagnosis if we continue to look only for compounds that stain with ninhydrin. I think that this is the beauty of this meeting. We are talking about different ways of detecting defects in metabolism which produce overwhelming illness in early life.

Watts (*Harrow*). Is it possible to use coenzyme A therapeutically in ketotic hyperglycinaemia?

The condensation product of glyoxylate and oxaloacetate inhibits the tricarboxylic acid cycle. Glyoxylate is closely related to glycine and an analogue of this type rather than homocitrate might be the toxic factor.

Does Dr Levin have any control values for his leucocyte enzymes in children as opposed to adults?

Further, does Dr Levin have information on the mechanism of action of the enzyme for which he is postulating two mutations, one involving the substrate binding site and the other the coenzyme binding site? The postulates could be tested by studying the kinetic behaviour of the enzyme.

Nyhan. I do not have any information on the administration of coenzyme A as a therapeutic manoeuvre. I do not feel that it is relevant to the fundamental defect, but it is conceivable that in some of these clinical situations in which there is an extreme degree of acidosis the symptomatology might be relevant to competition for the pool of co-enzyme A. This has not been our hypothesis, but it is a reasonable one and it suggests the experiment.

Levin (*London*). In reply to Dr Watts, we have so far only normal levels in adults. There are ethical difficulties in obtaining blood from normal children for this assay. Although it would have been possible to attempt to differentiate the two postulated variants of methylmalonyl CoA mutase by studying Km values, pH optima, etc., it would be difficult to undertake such studies using leucocyte homogenates because of the relatively large amounts of blood required. It would probably be simpler if liver were used. Furthermore, neither of the patients we examined were vitamin B_{12} dependent, so that we would not in any case have been able to compare results with the second variant.

Perry (*Vancouver*). Do untreated patients with methylmalonic aciduria have a characteristic odour to their breath, bodies or urine? Authentic samples of methylmalonic acid have a very distinctive odour.

Levin. In reply to Dr Perry, we have not observed any characteristic odour in these patients either in their breath, bodies or urine. It is not correct to say that authentic specimens of methylmalonic acid have a distinctive smell. Although some commercial preparations of the acid have an appreciable but not unpleasant odour, methylmalonic acid whether recrystallised from the commercial acid or obtained from the urine of these patients, is odourless.

Pennock (*Bristol*). What advice on simple screening techniques for these disorders could the speakers give? Should the onus of detecting these conditions rest with the clinician or with the laboratory staff who are often asked to screen for a whole range of diseases?

Levin. In reply to Dr Pennock, both clinicians and pathologists should have a high degree of suspicion in possible cases of inborn errors of metabolism in children. After direct paper chromatography of the urine, using butanol-acetic acid-water as the solvent system, the distal half of the dried paper is stained with bromcresolgreen. Any distinct yellow spot requires further investigation. For methylmalonic acid, a relatively simple colour reaction can be carried out on the urine (Oberholzer *et al*., 1967, *Arch. Dis. Childh*., **42**, 492).

Nyhan. Let me try the same question. I would certainly reiterate the previous comments. I would also like to speak for an uncertainty factor. It seems to me that we are just at the beginnings of defining good ways to screen. After all as I see it we have not yet really defined all the diseases that make up the organic acidaemias. We have not really established the extent of the different phenotypes one could look for, and it is probably only going to be then that we will be able to develop really good economical methods of screening.

At this point I would like to emphasize the importance of clinical screening that was brought up before—those of us who operate screening laboratories tend not to get samples from patients of the sort that we are talking about. We get samples from people who look odd, have mental retardation, and have seizures and many kinds of chronic illnesses, but we are not getting them from neonatal nurseries, from babies who are overwhelmingly ill or acidotic. Goodness knows, most of the time the baby who is acidotic in the new-born nursery is assumed to have lactic acidosis, and due to oxygen insufficiency. What I would recommend is that people begin looking for simple things in the newborn nursery. For instance, is the baby ketotic? Does he have ketones in the urine? Most of the time the neonatologist does not know this. If the infant does have ketosis and is a sick newborn, he is a candidate for this kind of screening.

In another kind of presentation, the baby is acidotic and there is an unexplained anion gap. This is a patient in whom one could begin to screen for organic acidaemia.

The other aspect of the uncertainty factor is that we are talking generally about volatile compounds which can readily disappear from blood and urine. It is therefore not easy to be sure, if we are simply screening for the organic acids, that we are going to find the abnormality we are looking for. Ideal methods of screening are in the process of being developed, rather than already being fully developed and merely awaiting widespread application.

Let me give a specific example. We have recently had experience with the diagnosis of isovaleric acidaemia. There is no question that if we had been looking for that patient by screening for isovaleric acid in the blood or the urine, we would never have found it. What we did discover was that isovalerylglycine is a major and consistent product of an excess of isovaleric acid. Subsequently we developed a screening method for the detection of acylglycine derivatives. This can be done very simply by using TLC. Our method was published in *Clinical Chemistry* (**16**, 420, 1970). Now we have a good method for screening for isovaleric acidaemia, whereas I do not think that existed before. Similar approaches to methodology may have to be developed for each of these organic acidaemias.

Curtius (*Zurich*). In a case of non-ketotic hyperglycinaemia we also found a high excretion of methylmalonic acid. In addition, however, we could see a number of other organic acids (e.g. benzoic, succinic, glycollic, 3-hydroxyisobutyric, lactic, propionic, isovaleric, valeric and isocaproic). How would you explain these results?

Levin. Apart from lactic, uric and acetic acids, the only organic acid we sought for or estimated in the urine of our patient was propionic acid, the precursor of methylmalonic acid. This was present in the urine to the extent of 95 mg per 24 hr., greatly in excess of the amount normally excreted, less than 0·5 mg per day. Such an increase is to be expected from the site of the metabolic block. We have not studied organic acid excretion by gas chromatography.

Black (*Sheffield*). Should we use tests for ketosis as screening methods? Unfortunately testing for acetonuria has fallen into disuse. What are the speakers' views on testing for acetonuria? Is the pattern of ketosis similar to that in diabetes?

Levin. The answer to the last question is yes, except there is no hyperglycaemia. I do not attach as much importance to ketosis as others have done. In ill children, ketosis as measured by urinary ketone tests is not infrequent and if all of them were screened for the organic acids involved, I am doubtful whether the success rate would be better than now. Ketosis is interesting in cases of methylmalonic aciduria, but from a diagnostic point of view it is only one factor and not the only finger of suspicion.

Nyhan. As a clinician you can distinguish between ketosis and more ketosis. Most children having ketosis on admission are put on parenteral fluid, and the next specimen has no ketones. No one has problems with that kind of case, and these represent close to 100 per cent of dehydrated children coming into the hospital.

The kind of case I am talking about is the one who sits about acidotic for several days, in whom, despite massive amounts of bicarbonate, the urine is still loaded with ketones. Nevertheless, unless you test urine for acetone, you will never find such a patient.

PROPIONIC ACIDAEMIA

by

D. GOMPERTZ

PROPIONIC acidaemia was first described as an inborn error of metabolism by Hommes and his colleagues in 1968. They described a child who died at the age of 5 days with severe hypotonia, areflexia, hyperventilation and grunting. This child had a severe metabolic acidosis which was resistant to therapy. This acidosis was due to the presence of a very high concentration of propionate in the blood (5·4 mmol). Hommes and his colleagues concluded that the most likely biochemical basis for this severe degree of propionic acidaemia was a decreased activity of propionyl CoA carboxylase (E.C. 6.4.1.3.). The accumulation of odd-numbered fatty acids in the child's tissues indicated a raised intracellular propionyl CoA concentration, providing further evidence that the enzyme block was associated with propionyl CoA carboxylase (Fig. 1).

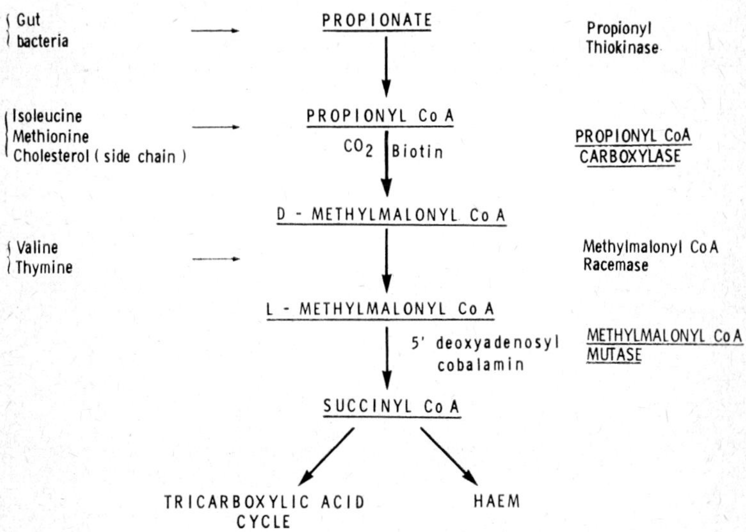

FIG. 1. Metabolism of propionic acid.

The second child with this condition presented 2 years later, with increasing apnoeic episodes, regurgitation of feeds and hypotonia (Gompertz *et al.*, 1970). An increasingly severe metabolic acidosis and ketosis prompted a search for an organic acidaemia and the child was found to have a plasma propionate of 2·5 mmol. The acidosis was resistant to therapy and the child died on the eighth day. A mitochondrial preparation isolated from the liver within an hour of death was used to establish the nature of the enzyme defect. This preparation showed a propionyl CoA carboxylase activity of less than 10 per cent of normal, with a normal methylmalonyl CoA mutase activity (E.C. 5.4.99.2.).

Both of these children had elevated concentrations of several amino acids in the plasma. Lysine, histidine, valine, isoleucine and leucine were raised in both children, but a high glycine concentration (1·00 mmol) was only found in the second child. This pattern of plasma amino acids appeared characteristic of ketotic hyperglycinaemia and analysis of the urine by gas-liquid chromatography demonstrated the presence of long-chain ketones.

Ketotic hyperglycinaemia was first described in 1961 by Childs, Nyhan, Borden, Bard and Cooke. The clinical syndrome consists of persistent vomiting with ketosis, acidosis and lethargy. Extensive studies were performed to establish the cause of the hyperglycinaemia but the basic enzyme defects associated with this condition remained obscure until 1967. Then Stokke and colleagues described a child with methylmalonic acidaemia, presenting in the neonatal period with a clinical picture of a severe metabolic acidosis. Plasma amino acid analysis revealed increased concentrations of glycine and lysine and this led Stokke *et al.* to comment on the clinical and biochemical similarities of methylmalonic acidaemia and ketotic hyperglycinaemia. This interrelationship has been described since by several groups (Morrow *et al.*, 1969) and it is now established that although methylmalonyl CoA mutase deficiency may present with the clinical picture of the 'ketotic hyperglycinaemia syndrome', the hyperglycinaemia may be transient and the ketosis is not always present.

The relationship between propionyl CoA carboxylase deficiency and the 'ketotic hyperglycinaemia syndrome' had already been suspected for some time. Hsia, Scully and Rosenberg (1969) were investigating methylmalonic acid metabolism in an affected 6-year-old sister of the first patient with ketotic hyperglycinaemia described by Childs and his associates. They demonstrated that peripheral leucocytes from this child were unable to oxidise ^{14}C-propionate to carbon dioxide although ^{14}C-methylmalonate was oxidised normally. This suggested a metabolic block in the formation of methylmalonyl CoA from propionate, probably an impairment of the activity of propionyl CoA carboxylase. Subsequently, Hsia and his colleagues (1971), using cultured fibroblasts, demonstrated that the metabolic block in this child was a deficient propionyl CoA carboxylase activity.

These demonstrations, both in a neonate and in a 6-year-old child, of the identity of propionyl CoA carboxylase deficiency and the 'ketotic hyperglycinaemia syndrome' have prompted a reassessment of existing children known to have this syndrome. After the initial suggestion that methylmalonic acidaemia and ketotic hyperglycinaemia were identical, all the existing children known to have ketotic hyperglycinaemia were investigated for methylmalonic acidaemia. Two children at Great Ormond Street Hospital, London, with ketotic hyperglycinaemia have now been re-investigated and shown to have propionic acidaemia. These children had been maintained carefully on low-protein diets and had survived numerous acidotic episodes in infancy. However, the extent of the impairment of their propionyl CoA carboxylase activities must have been very much less than in the two initial cases of neonatal propionic acidaemia described earlier. We found the plasma concentrations of propionate only rose to 0·6 and 0·16 mmol respectively after isoleucine loading tests (Barnes *et al.*, 1970). This suggested that these children are suffering from a variant of the original condition and led to a trial of biotin, the prosthetic group for propionyl CoA carboxylase. Treatment with biotin (5 mg b.d.) modified the response of one of these children to an isoleucine loading test (Barnes *et al.*, 1970). The plasma propionate increased to a much lesser extent and the child did not show ketonuria in response to the isoleucine load. Treatment with biotin made little difference to the clinical status of this child, but recently Dr Y. E. Hsia has observed a clinical improvement in one child after biotin therapy (personal communication).

Hommes and his colleagues reported that an elder sibling of their case died with identical symptoms some years previously although the parents had had three other healthy children. A sibling of the second case (Gompertz *et al.*, 1970) also died with similar symptoms and a gas-liquid chromatographic tracing of this child's plasma long-chain fatty acids performed during life showed the presence of odd-numbered fatty acids, establishing the diagnosis in retrospect. The parents in this case were first cousins and other first cousin marriages in this family had given rise to similar neonatal deaths. The child that Hsia *et al.* (1969) have studied is a sister of the first child with ketotic hyperglycinaemia documented by Childs *et al.* (1961), and the parents of these children have intermediate levels of the enzyme (Hsia *et al.*, 1971). The occurrence of this condition within various sibships, the inheritance pattern demonstrated by the second case and the intermediate levels of enzyme in parents, indicates an autosomal recessive mode of inheritance.

The dietary management of children with ketotic hyperglycinaemia was empirical. Early studies had established which amino acids are especially ketogenic (Childs & Nyhan, 1964) and the children have since been maintained on as low-protein diet as possible. The demonstration that propionyl CoA carboxylase and methylmalonyl CoA mutase deficiencies are responsible for this clinical picture does not help to rationalise dietary treatment. The propionate-methylmalonate pathway links the degradation of valine, isoleucine (Gompertz, Jones & Knowles, 1967) the side-chain of cholesterol (Mitropoulos, Myant & Gompertz, 1970) and perhaps polyunsaturated fatty acids (Dupont & Mathias, 1969) to the tricarboxylic acid cycle, and is also responsible for handling the load of propionate produced by gut bacteria (Williams & Spray, 1970). Other metabolites also contribute to this pathway, but their quantitative importance is in doubt. It has been assumed that odd-numbered fatty acids are a major source of propionate, but there is little evidence that there is significant absorption of these acids from the intestine. The numerous sources of propionate or propionyl CoA make dietary modification difficult to rationalise.

Propionyl CoA carboxylase is a biotin enzyme and in common with other carboxylases requires a ligase to attach biotin to the apo-enzyme (Seigel, Foote & Coon, 1965). Biotin itself requires activation via its adenylate prior to attachment to its apo-enzyme (Seigel *et al.*, 1965). Recent studies of acetyl CoA carboxylase in biotin-deficient and supplemented rats demonstrate that there is normally a proportion of catalytically inactive apo-enzyme not containing biotin (Jacobs, Kilburn & Majerus, 1970). The requirements for activation of biotin and for an apo-enzyme-biotin ligase and the possibility of free apo-enzyme present in tissues normally, may lead to a number of biochemical variants of impaired propionyl CoA carboxylases that might respond to biotin. The demonstration of a raised plasma propionate should always be followed by a trial of biotin therapy as previous experience with other cases of propionic acidaemia is no guide to the possibility of biotin-responsiveness.

The clinical presentation of the 'ketotic hyperglycinaemia syndrome' is difficult to explain even now that the basic enzyme defects are known. Inhibition of enzymes acting on co-enzyme A esters will undoubtedly cause a far-reaching redistribution of free and esterified co-enzyme A levels in each cellular compartment. Menkes (1966) suggested that the long-chain ketones produced in this condition are formed from β keto-acids that are usually present as their co-enzyme A esters; the free acids probably decarboxylate spontaneously to produce the long-chain ketones.

The problem of hyperglycinaemia is more difficult to explain. Studies of glycine metabolism in children with ketotic hyperglycinaemia have failed to reveal a defect in glycine degradation. Perhaps the most important clue to the mechanism of the hyperglycinaemia comes from a comparison of propionic, methylmalonic and isovaleric acidaemias and β-methylcrotonyl glycinuria. The first two conditions may give hyperglycinaemia, in isovaleric acidaemia in remission the isovaleric acid is excreted as the glycine conjugate (Tanaka & Isselbacher, 1967) and in methylcrotonyl glycinuria the free acid does not appear in the urine (Eldjarn *et al.*, 1970). The occurrence of the glycine conjugates of these aliphatic acids in these conditions appears to parallel the specificity of the mitochondrial enzyme, glycine-N-acylase (Schachter & Taggart, 1954). It might be suggested that these increased acyl CoA concentrations in the mitochondrial compartment induce an increased glycine production. In those conditions in which the acyl groups do not conjugate, i.e. in propionic and methylmalonic acidaemias, the excess glycine produced would spill out into the circulation.

Acknowledgements

It is a pleasure to thank Professor C. C. Booth and numerous other colleagues for their advice and helpful suggestions regarding topics included in this article. I am also grateful to the Medical Research Council and the National Fund for Research into Crippling Disease for financial support.

REFERENCES

BARNES, N. D., HULL, D., BALGOBIN, L. & GOMPERTZ, D. (1970) *Lancet*, **i**, 244.
CHILDS, B. & NYHAN, W. L. (1964) *Pediatrics*, **33**, 403.
CHILDS, B., NYHAN, W. L., BORDEN, M., BARD, L. & COOKE, R. E. (1961) *Pediatrics*, **27**, 522.
DUPONT, J. & MATHIAS, M. M. (1969) *Lipids*, **4**, 6.
ELDJARN, L., JELLUM, E., STOKKE, O., PANDE, H. & WAALER, P. E. (1970) *Lancet*, **ii**, 521.
GOMPERTZ, D., JONES, J. H. & KNOWLES, J. P. (1967) *Clin. chim. Acta*. **18**, 197.
GOMPERTZ, D., STORRS, C. N., BAU, D. C. K., PETERS, T. J. & HUGHES, E. A. (1970) *Lancet*, **i**, 1140.
HOMMES, F. A., KUIPERS, J. R. G., ELEMA, J. D., JANSEN, J. F. & JONXIS, J. H. P. (1968) *Pediat. Res.*, **2**, 519.
HSIA, Y. E., SCULLY, K. J. & ROSENBERG, L. E. (1969) *Lancet*, **i**, 757.
HSIA, Y. E., SCULLY, K. J. & ROSENBERG, L. E. (1971) *J. clin. Invest.*, **50**, 127.
JACOBS, R., KILBURN, E. & MAJERUS, P. W. (1970) *J. biol. Chem.*, **245**, 6462.
MENKES, J. H. (1966) *J. Pediat.*, **69**, 413.
MITROPOULOS, K. A., MYANT, N. B. & GOMPERTZ, D. (1970) *Biochem. J.*, **118**, 551.
MORROW, G.III., BARNESS, L. A., AUERBACH, V. H., DIGEORGE, A. M., ANDO, T. & NYHAN, W. L. (1969) *J. Pediat.*, **74**, 680.
NYHAN, W. L., BORDEN, M. & CHILDS, B. (1961) *Pediatrics*, **27**, 539.
SCHACHTER, D. & TAGGART, J. V. (1954) *J. biol. Chem.*, **208**, 263.
SIEGEL, L., FOOTE, J. L. & COON, M. J. (1965) *J. biol. Chem.*, **240**, 1025.
STOKKE, O., ELDJARN, L., NORUM, K. R., STEEN-JOHNSON, J. & HALVORSEN, S. (1967) *Scand. J. clin. Lab. Invest.*, **20**, 313.
TANAKA, K. & ISSELBACHER, K. J. (1967) *J. biol. Chem.*, **242**, 2966.
WILLIAMS, D. L. & SPRAY, G. H. (1970) *Brit. J. Nutr.*, **24**, 204.

DISCUSSION
(of paper by Dr. Gompertz)

Nyhan (*La Jolla*). Propionyl glycine has now been identified in the urine of a patient with ketotic hyperglycinaemia and propionic acidaemia (unpublished data). This is not in agreement with Dr Gompertz' hypothesis.

Gompertz (*London*). Propionyl glycine excretion does not regularly occur in propionic acidaemia, and when it does it is only in trace amounts. The excretion of isovaleryl glycine in isovaleric acidaemia may be between 0·5 and 1·5 g per day and β-methylcrotonyl glycine and tiglyl glycine excretion in β-methylcrotonyl glycinuria may exceed 200 mg per day. The trace amounts of propionyl glycine (less than 10 mg per 24 hours) indicate clearly that the conjugation of propionyl CoA and glycine does not occur to any great extent and that there may be a relationship between this failure of conjugation and the hyperglycinaemia found in this condition.

A NEW METABOLIC ERROR IN THE LEUCINE DEGRADATION PATHWAY: β-HYDROXYISOVALERIC ACIDURIA AND β-METHYLCROTONYLGLYCINURIA

by

ODDVAR STOKKE, EGIL JELLUM AND LORENTZ ELDJARN

UNTIL now two different inborn errors of metabolism have been found in the degradative pathway of leucine, viz. maple syrup urine disease and isovaleric acidaemia. Recently we (Eldjarn, Jellum, Stokke, Pande & Waaler, 1970; Stokke, Eldjarn, Jellum, Pande & Waaler, 1972) have come across a third defect in this pathway, characterised by excretion of substantial amounts of β-hydroxyisovaleric acid (β-OH-IV) and β-methylcrotonyl glycine (β-MCG) in the urine.

Case history

The patient was a 4½ months old girl, whose mother and father's mother were first cousins. Two elder brothers of the child are healthy. Pregnancy and delivery were normal, and the child appeared well at birth. Right from the second week of life, however, there were feeding difficulties. Gradually she revealed signs of retarded motor developments, muscular hypotonia and muscular atrophy. The deep tendon reflexes could not be elicited, and fibrillation of the tongue was seen. Growth was normal, but the weight gain rather slow. The clinical picture resembled that of a progressive infantile spinal muscular atrophy (Werdnig-Hoffmann's disease). In addition, however, the urine had an unpleasant smell, like that of cat's urine. There were no signs of other diseases, especially no clinical signs of biotin deficiency and no acidotic episodes. Mental development seemed to be normal.

Laboratory findings

By our screening procedure for metabolic disorders, using gas-liquid chromatography (GLC) and mass spectrometry (MS) (Jellum, Stokke & Eldjarn, 1971), large amounts of two abnormal metabolites were found in the child's urine (Fig. 1). These two compounds were shown to be β-hydroxyisovaleric acid (β-OH-IV) and β-methylcrotonyl glycine (β-MCG). The child excreted about 400 mg per day of the former substance and about 100 mg per day of the latter. Our GLC-method did not detect either of these metabolites or any abnormal accumulation of short-chain fatty acids (including isovaleric acid) in the blood. The concentration of these compounds in serum must therefore be below 0·5 mg/100 ml, which is the sensitivity limit of the method.

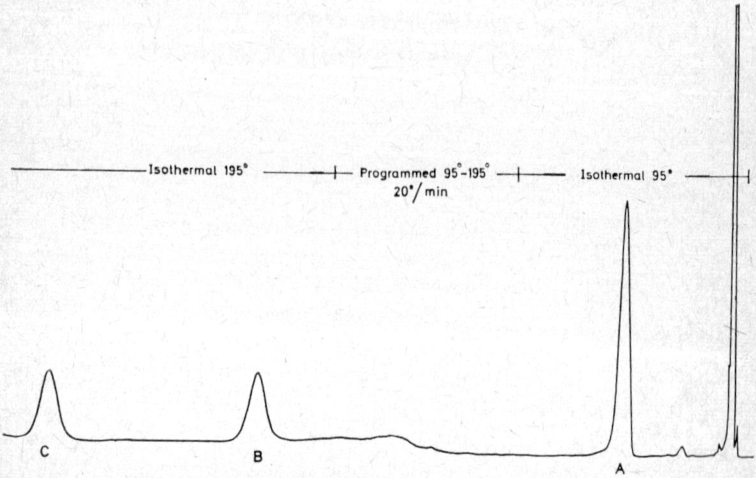

FIG. 1. Gas liquid chromatogram of the methylated acids from the patient's urine. The first-eluted peak represents β-hydroxy-isovaleric acid, the second peak β-methylcrotonyl glycine and the third hippuric acid.

Examination of the amino acids by GLC showed a normal pattern in the urine, and only slight elevations of some of the serum amino acids, including leucine. The daily excretion of creatinine in the urine showed only small variations, with an average of 30 mg. The excretion of creatine was about 80 mg per day at 6 months of age; during the next 2 months it decreased slowly to about 50 mg.

Interpretation of findings

The excretion of β-OH-IV and β-MCG is most probably caused by an enzyme defect in the degradation of leucine. The normal degradation of leucine proceeds as follows (Fig. 2). After transamination, oxidative decarboxylation and dehydrogenation, leucine is converted to β-methylcrotonyl CoA. By a biotin-dependent CO_2 fixation this acid is converted to β-methylglutaconyl CoA, which is further metabolised to β-hydroxy-β-methylglutaryl CoA. This acid is split, to form acetoacetate and acetyl CoA.

A block in the CO_2 fixation mechanism, which is the most likely cause of the metabolic failure in our patient, would primarily lead to an intracellular accumulation of β-methylcrotonyl CoA. It was shown some

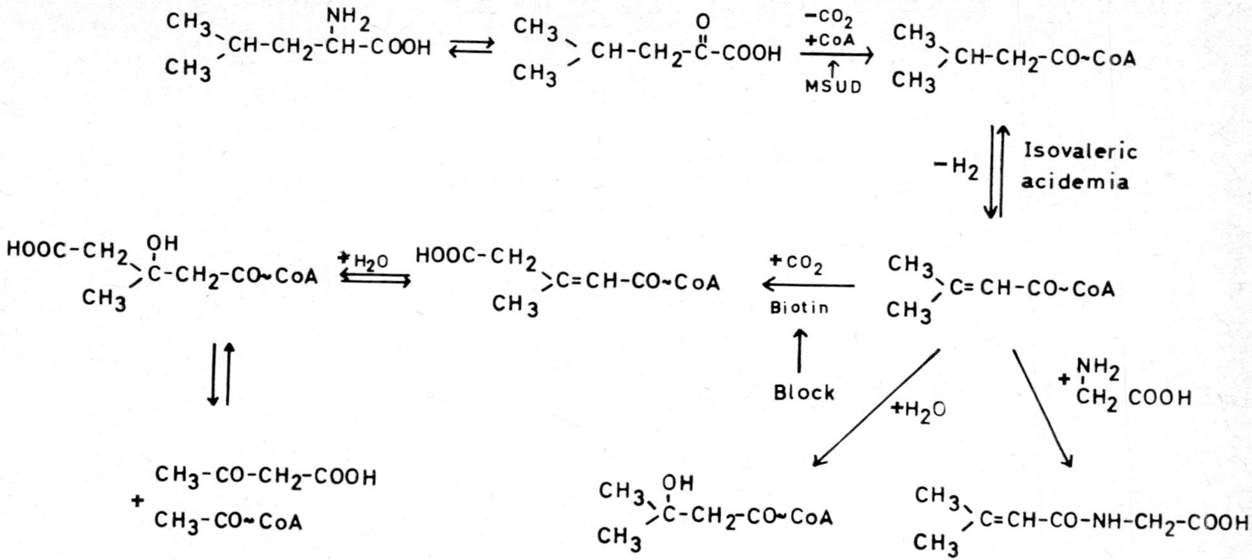

FIG. 2. The degradative pathway of leucine. The probable block in our patient and the defects in maple syrup urine disease (MSUD) and isovaleric acidaemia are indicated.

years ago that this compound can be metabolised to β-OH-IV, which in fact for some time was considered to be an obligatory intermediate in the degradation of leucine (Coon, Robinson & Bachhawat, 1955).

β-MCG is most likely formed by a conjugation of β-methylcrotonyl CoA with glycine. Conjugates between glycine and several short-chain fatty acids are well known to occur (Schachter & Taggart, 1954), and the mechanism probably parallels that forming hippuric acid from benzoyl CoA and glycine.

The amino acid chromatograms of the serum showed slight elevations of leucine and a few other amino acids. These elevations were, however, too small to be of any special significance. It should be noted that the oxidative decarboxylation of α-ketoisocaproic acid, leading to the formation of isovaleryl CoA, represents an irreversible step. Thus, accumulation of lower intermediates should not influence the concentration of leucine.

Neither β-OH-IV nor β-MCG have the peculiar smell present in the urine from the patient. We cannot give any exact explanation of this odour. However, both β-methylcrotonic acid and isovaleric acid smell like cat's urine, and the smell is very strong and penetrating. It may be that the smell of the urine is caused by small and not detectable amounts of β-methylcrotonic acid and isovaleric acid.

Clinically as well as biochemically this new disorder is distinctly different from those previously described in the leucine pathway. Both maple syrup urine disease (MSUD) and isovaleric acidaemia are characterised by metabolic acidosis, central neurological manifestations with convulsions, rigidity, hyperreflexia, ataxia and mental disturbances. None of these symptoms could be found in our child. MSUD is caused by a defect in the oxidative decarboxylation of the α-keto acids derived from leucine, isoleucine and valine (for ref. see Dancis & Levitz, 1966). Both the three amino acids and their corresponding α-keto acids can be detected in high concentrations in blood and urine. Isovaleric acidaemia is due to a defective isovaleryl CoA dehydrogenase, leading to accumulation of isovaleric acid in blood and urine (Tanaka, Budd, Efron & Isselbacher, 1966). In addition two other metabolites, isovaleryl glycine and β-OH-IV, can be demonstrated in the urine (Tanaka & Isselbacher, 1967; Tanaka, Orr & Isselbacher, 1968). Although similar with respect to the urinary content of β-OH-IV, our patient did not excrete isovaleryl glycine, and β-MCG is not excreted in isovaleric acidaemia. The mechanism by which β-OH-IV is formed in the patients with isovaleric acidaemia is obscure, as the metabolic block is located prior to β-methylcrotonyl CoA. The hypothesis has been put forward that isovaleric acid is hydroxylated to β-OH-IV by an ω-oxidation mechanism (Tanaka, Orr & Isselbacher, 1968).

Treatment

The probability of a failure in the leucine degradation prompted us to try dietary treatment. The patient was given a diet containing the minimum requirement of leucine (about 150 mg leucine per kg body weight per day). Simultaneously she was given an extra supply of biotin, 250 μg per day, based on the optimistic hypothesis that this might increase the effectiveness of the β-methylcrotonyl CoA carboxylase. It should be noted that the biotin supply represented substitutional rather than therapeutic doses. Upon this treatment there occurred a rapid drop in the urinary excretion of β-OH-IV, from 400 mg to below 50 mg per day, and later on the quantity excreted paralleled the intake of leucine (Fig. 3). The changes

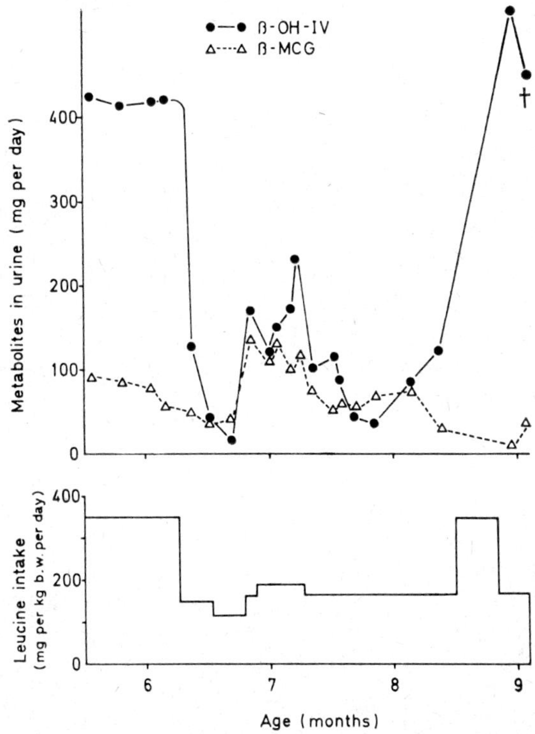

FIG. 3. Urinary excretion of β-hydroxyisovaleric acid and β-methyl-crotonyl glycine during the low-leucine treatment.

in the excretion of β-MCG were less pronounced. After having kept the patient on this treatment for over 2 months, she was given an ordinary diet for 1 week. The excretion of β-OH-IV was increased considerably by this change, reaching pre-treatment values. The daily biotin supply had been maintained during this week. It seems therefore likely that the decrease in excretion of metabolites following the treatment was an effect of the diet, and not of the biotin supply.

However, the child's clinical condition did not improve, in spite of treatment for several months. On the contrary, the symptoms got worse, and she died from bronchopneumonia at the age of 9 months. Permission for necropsy was refused by the parents.

Connection Between Biochemical Findings and Clinical Symptoms

We were unable to find any clinical improvement with the dietary treatment. One reason for this might be that the treatment was started too late, and that the neurological changes which had already occurred were irreversible. Another possibility is that the child actually was suffering from two independent disorders, one responsible for the clinical picture and the other responsible for the excretion of the metabolites. Based on one case only, it is impossible to draw any definite conclusions as to these questions. A patient with two rare disorders of possibly genetic origin is unusual, but the fact that the parents were consanguineous increases the chances of such a possibility. Up till now we have analysed the urine from six patients with progressive infantile spinal muscular atrophy for the accumulation of β-OH-IV and β-MCG, but so far none has been found.

None of the metabolites could be detected in the serum of the patient, which means that the concentration was well below 0·5 mg/100 ml. The renal clearance for these compounds must therefore be very high. With a daily excretion of β-OH-IV of about 400 mg, the clearance was at least five times that of creatinine. (The daily excretion of creatinine averaged 30 mg, and the serum level was 0·2-0·3 mg/100 ml.) This implies that an active renal excretion must take place and/or that a large part of the urinary β-OH-IV is produced in the kidneys.

In order to obtain additional information about the metabolic defect we cultured fibroblasts from a skin biopsy of the patient (Stokke & Lie, unpublished results). Two different growth media were used for the subcultures, one containing ample amounts of biotin (TC 199, Difco) supplemented with 20 per cent human serum and 10 per cent chick embryo extract, the other containing no biotin (Eagle's minimal medium, Difco) supplemented with 2 per cent serum and chick embryo extract. On the latter medium the cells survived only 1 week. After addition of (1-^{14}C) isovaleric acid (final concentration 10^{-4} mol/1) to the growth medium, the production of $^{14}CO_2$ was measured. We could then show that fibroblasts from our patient had equal ability to degrade isovaleric acid to CO_2 as had fibroblasts from two healthy controls. About 0·4-0·5 per cent of the added isovaleric acid was degraded per mg of fibroblast protein per hour, independent of the reduction in the biotin content of the growth medium.

Thus, we were unable to demonstrate any metabolic defects in the fibroblasts from the patient.

Theoretically, isovaleric acid may be degraded by two alternative routes, in addition to the ordinary pathway involving CO_2 fixation. Isovaleric acid may be ω-oxidised, to form α-methylsuccinic acid, which can then be further degraded by β-oxidation. Such a mechanism has been described for several other branched-chain fatty acids (for ref. see Eldjarn, Try & Stokke, 1966). α-Oxidation has been shown to be an alternative pathway for the degradation of β-methyl-substituted fatty acids in man (Stokke, Try & Eldjarn, 1967); the degradation of β-methylvaleric acid, which structurally is close to isovaleric acid, is initiated by an α-oxidation (Stokke, 1969). However, neither ω-oxidation nor α-oxidation seem to play any important role in the degradation of isovaleric acid, since they are not sufficiently effective to prevent accumulation of isovaleric acid in patients when the main pathway is blocked. The normal amounts of $^{14}CO_2$ produced from (1-^{14}C) isovaleric acid in the fibroblasts of our patients are therefore most likely explained by a degradation via CO_2 fixation. Thus, the defect in our patient with β-hydroxyisovaleric aciduria and β-methylcrotonyl glycinuria does not seem to be generalised.

Conclusions

The excretion of β-OH-IV and β-MCG in our patient was probably caused by a defective β-methylcrotonyl CoA carboxylase (E.C.6.4.1.4.). The drastic reduction of the urinary metabolites which was achieved by dietary treatment did not influence the clinical course. The renal clearance of β-OH-IV, and β-MCG must be very high, several times that of creatinine, indicating production in the kidney. Cultures of skin fibroblasts from the patient were able to degrade isovaleric acid to CO_2 at a normal rate. Based on these findings it is tempting to postulate that our patient suffered from two independent disorders, one causing the progressive neurological symptoms and the other leading to the excretion of β-OH-IV and β-MCG. The latter metabolic failure was probably located to the kidneys. Any definite conclusions must await discovery of other patients with β-hydroxyisovaleric aciduria and β-methylcrotonyl glycinuria.

References

Coon, M. J., Robinson, W. G. & Bachhawat, B. K. (1955) *In* McElroy, W. D. and Glass, B. (eds.). *A Symposium on Amino Acid Metabolism*, Baltimore: The Johns Hopkins Press, pp. 431–41.

Dancis, J. & Levitz, M. (1966) *In* Stanbury, J. B., Wyngaarden, J. B. and Fredrickson, D. S. (eds.). *The Metabolic Basis of Inherited Disease*, New York: McGraw-Hill, pp. 353–65.

ELDJARN, L., JELLUM, E., STOKKE, O., PANDE, H. & WAALER, P. E. (1970) *Lancet*, ii, 521.

JELLUM, E., STOKKE, O. & ELDJARN, L. (1971) *Scand. J. clin. Lab. Invest.*, **27**, 273.

ELDJARN, L., TRY, K. & STOKKE, O. (1966) *Scand. J. clin. Lab. Invest.*, **18**, 141.

SCHACHTER, D. & TAGGART, J. V. (1954) *J. biol. Chem.*, **208**, 263.

STOKKE, O. (1969) *Biochim. biophys. Acta*, **176**, 54.

STOKKE, O., ELDJARN, L., JELLUM, E., PANDE, H., WAALER, P. E., (1972) *Pediatrics*, **49**, 726.

STOKKE, O., TRY, K. & ELDJARN, L. (1967) *Biochim. biophys. Acta*, **144**, 271.

TANAKA, K., BUDD, M. A., EFRON, M. L. & ISSELBACHER, K. J. (1966) *Proc. nat. Acad. Sci. (Wash.)*, **56**, 236.

TANAKA, K. & ISSELBACHER, K. J. (1967) *J. biol. Chem.*, **242**, 2966.

TANAKA, K., ORR, J. C. & ISSELBACHER, K. J. (1968) *Biochim. biophys. Acta*, **152**, 638.

TIGLYL GLYCINE EXCRETION IN A CHILD WITH β-METHYLCROTONYL GLYCINURIA

by

D. GOMPERTZ AND G. H. DRAFFAN

ELDJARN and his colleagues (1970) have described a child with β-methylcrotonyl glycinuria and β-hydroxyisovaleric aciduria, presumably due to an impaired β-methylcrotonyl CoA carboxylase activity. We have recently studied a further child with these abnormal metabolites in his urine. This communication describes the identification of a third abnormal metabolite present in the urine in large amounts, as tiglyl glycine.

The first indication that this child has β-methylcrotonyl glycinuria was the detection of β-methylcrotonic acid as the free acid by gas-chromatography on a neopentylglycoladipate-phosphoric acid column after the steam distillation of urine. Subsequent experiments showed that the acid conditions used for steam distillation were sufficient for hydrolysis of β-methylcrotonyl glycine. The next procedure was to extract the urine with diethyl ether and to analyse the methylated extract for the glycine conjugate of β-methylcrotonic acid. Heptadecanoic acid was added to the ether extract prior to methylation with diazomethane. Gas chromatography on a 15 per cent diethylene glycol succinate column at 175° revealed two large abnormal peaks with retention times of 2·97 and 3·31 relative to heptadecanoic acid. The second and larger peak (Rt 3.31) had a retention time identical to a sample of authenticated β-methylcrotonyl glycine kindly provided by Dr Jellum and Professor Eldjarn, Institute of Clinical Biochemistry, Oslo. Analysis of these peaks on an A.E.I. M.S.12 mass spectrometer coupled to a gas-chromatograph showed identity of mass spectra between the peak in this child's urine (Rt 3·31) and β-methylcrotonyl glycinemethyl ester in the sample from Professor Eldjarn's department.

The first peak (Rt 2·97) had a similar but not identical mass spectrum to β-methylcrotonyl glycine methyl ester, suggesting that it might be an isomer. Early studies of leucine degradation had been concerned with the possibility that β-methylvinylacetyl CoA might be an intermediate in this pathway and an enzyme, β-methylvinylacetyl CoA isomerase has been described that converts β-methylvinylacetyl CoA to β-methylcrotonyl CoA in ox liver (Rilling & Coon, 1960). It seemed possible that this second peak might be the glycine conjugate of β-methylvinylacetyl CoA, i.e. a double bond isomer of β-methylcrotonyl glycine. In order to investigate this possibility, the two peaks (Rt 2·97 & 3·31) were collected separately and hydrogenated over a palladium-charcoal catalyst. The β-methylcrotonyl glycine peak after hydrogenation gave a material with identical retention time and mass spectrum to synthetic isovaleryl glycine methyl ester made by the method of Bondi and Eissler (1916). However, the first peak (Rt 2·97) gave a material with a different retention time and mass spectrum, thus excluding β-methylvinylacetyl glycine as a possible structure.

The collected material from the first peak was then hydrolysed in an attempt to identify the acyl group as the free acid on a neopentylglycol adipate column. Acid hydrolysis gave a peak with the same retention time as tiglic acid (α-methylcrotonic acid). Tiglyl glycine was then synthesised by a modification of the method of Bondi and Eissler and was isolated from the reaction mixture by preparative t.l.c., (silica gel H-chloroform, methanol, formic acid 92:7:1 by volume). The retention time of the methyl ester of the synthetic tiglyl glycine and its mass spectrum were identical to those of the first peak. The mass spectrum of the hydrogenated material was consistent with α-methylbutyryl glycine methyl ester.

The response of the gas-chromatograph detector to β-methylcrotonyl glycine was established by measuring the β-methylcrotonyl glycine peak before and after hydrogenation and comparing it with heptadecanoic acid. The response of synthetic isovaleryl glycine relative to heptadecanoic acid was established at the same time. The detector response to tiglyl glycine was assumed to be the same as β-methylcrotonyl glycine and this data was used to measure daily excretion levels of the two conjugates. Immediately after admission, the patient excreted similar amounts of both conjugates but after a week on a negligible protein intake, the tiglyl glycine excretion fell to less than one-tenth of the β-methylcrotonyl glycine excretion.

Tiglyl CoA is an intermediate on the isoleucine degradation pathway and is converted by enoyl hydratase to α-methyl β-hydroxybutyryl CoA. Tiglyl CoA and β-methylcrotonyl CoA are positional isomers and it seems likely that a raised intracellular concentration of β-methylcrotonyl CoA might inhibit the metabolism of tiglyl CoA resulting in the excretion of tiglyl glycine. The clinical and biochemical response of this child to biotin (Gompertz *et al*., 1971) indicates that the primary lesion was in the metabolism of β-methylcrotonyl CoA rather than tiglyl CoA. β-Methylcrotonyl CoA, unlike tiglyl CoA, requires a biotin-dependent carboxylation for its breakdown.

Acknowledgements

We are grateful to Professors C. C. Booth and C. T. Dollery for their interest and encouragement during this investigation and to Drs Hull and Watts for their clinical collaboration. The Medical Research Council and the National Fund for Research into Crippling Diseases are thanked for generous financial support.

REFERENCES

BONDI, S. & EISSLER, F. (1916) *Biochem. Z.*, **23**, 499.
ELDJARN, L., JELLUM, E., STOKKE, O., PANDE, H. & WAALER, P. E. (1970) *Lancet*, **ii**, 521.
GOMPERTZ, D., DRAFFAN, G. H., WATTS, J. L. & HULL, D. (1971) *Lancet*, **ii**, 22.
RILLING, H. C. & COON, M. J. (1960) *J. biol. Chem.*, **235**, 3087.

DISCUSSION
(of papers by Dr Stokke and Dr Gompertz)

Stokke (*Oslo*). The clinical symptoms of Dr Gompertz's patient and of our Norwegian child are completely different. Biochemically our patient excreted β-hydroxyisovaleric acid as the major metabolite and lesser amounts of β-methylcrotonyl glycine. Dr Gompertz's patient excreted β-methylcrotonyl glycine as the major metabolite, lesser amounts of β-hydroxyisovaleric acid, and in addition also tiglyl glycine. The response of the two patients to biotin was also different. Both patients were probably suffering from a defect in β-methylcrotonyl CoA carboxylase. In my opinion, we are dealing with two variants of the same disease, the two patients being another example of genetic heterogeneity in an inborn error of metabolism.

Gompertz (*London*). The biochemical and clinical symptomatology of these two patients will depend on the relative rates of the alternative enzymes acting upon β-methylcrotonyl CoA. The relative amounts of β-methylcrotonyl glycine and β-hydroxyisovaleric acid excreted will be a reflection of the competition of the enzymes enoyl hydratase and glycine-N-acylase for β-methylcrotonyl CoA as a substrate. The intracellular concentration of β-methylcrotonyl CoA will also depend on the activities of these two enzymes. We suggest that in our case the ketosis was secondary to a diminished availability of free co-enzyme A due to a high intercellular β-methylcrotonyl CoA concentration.

Cusworth (*London*). If the patient still excretes both metabolites I would suggest selective restriction of dietary intake of leucine and isoleucine. If tiglic acid production is the primary defect then dietary restriction of isoleucine could lead to disappearance of tiglic acid, and if this is the primary defect, also to disappearance of β-methylcrotonyl glycine. If, however, tiglic acid excretion is secondary then the β-methylcrotonyl glycine excretion would persist in spite of reduced isoleucine intake.

Gompertz. The Norwegian patient has unfortunately died and our patient no longer excretes these metabolites.

Curtius (*Zurich*). I would suggest the use of a nitrogen-sensitive detector for the more specific detection of glycine conjugates.

Gompertz. We find the flame ionisation detector still the most useful detector for a whole range of urinary metabolites.

Stokke. A nitrogen-sensitive detector for the glycine conjugates and other N-containing substances may make the gas-chromatograms somewhat easier to interpret, but you still have to identify the compounds. The use of mass spectrometry has, however, made the need for a nitrogen-sensitive detector very small.

Watts (*Harrow*). How unstable are these compounds on steam distillation? What is the recovery of the glycine conjugates and corresponding unconjugated compounds on ether extraction?

Stokke. Steam distillation after acidification may give rise to several artefacts, which must be born in mind. Conjugates, such as β-methylcrotonyl glycine and isovaleryl glycine, may be split. β-hydroxyisovaleric acid will split off water upon heating at low pH. Both β-hydroxyisovaleric acid and β-methylcrotonyl glycine are very water-soluble, making it time-consuming to get at quantitative extraction with diethyl ether. In our quantitative studies, therefore, we used methyl acetate. Extraction four times with two volumes of methyl acetate will give a 95–97 per cent yield.

Gompertz. These glycine conjugates are hydrolysed to a small extent during steam distillation and this accounted for our finding β-methylcrotonic acid in our child's urine while screening for volatile fatty acids. β-Methylcrotonyl and tiglyl glycine are not fully extracted into diethyl ether by hand-extraction methods but continuous liquid/liquid extraction of the urine overnight ensures quantitative recovery.

Nyhan (*La Jolla*). Tiglic acid and tiglyl glycine but no methylcrotonic acid or methylcrotonyl glycine were found in the urine of two patients with propionic acidaemia and ketotic hyperglycinaemia. Our hypothesis is that propionyl CoA accumulates much faster than acrylyl CoA and that there is competition for crotonase (enoyl hydratase). This would suggest that tiglyl glycine is the result of a secondary block.

Gompertz. Analysis of urine samples from five children with propionic acidaemia has shown us that the excretion of trace amounts of several other organic acids always occurs in this condition. This is no doubt due to the inhibitory effect of propionyl CoA on various other enzyme systems using coenzyme A esters as substrates. It is important to distinguish this type of effect from the major interaction between two similar biochemical pathways that we have suggested to account for the excessive excretion of tiglyl glycine in our case of β-methylcrotonyl glycinuria.

Eldjarn (*Oslo*). I should like to return to the fact that in Dr Gompertz's patient, treatment with 10 mg per day of biotin for several days led to the disappearance of the pathological metabolites from the urine. In our patient doses of only 0·25 mg per day were used. I understand from Dr Gompertz that stopping the biotin for a few days did not lead to the reappearance of the metabolites. This raises the question of the half-life of the biotin-dependent CO_2 fixing enzyme, since we know that the biotin is firmly ligated to the apo-enzymes by an amide bond. Most probably each of the many biotin-dependent enzymes has its own half-life, which may be weeks or even months. For ethical reasons it may, therefore, prove to be out of the question to re-establish the pathological excretion pattern in the patient's urine.

FURTHER STUDIES ON LEIGH'S ENCEPHALOMYELOPATHY

by

C. J. de Groot, J. H. P. Jonxis and F. A. Hommes

Subacute necrotising encephalomyelopathy or Leigh's disease is a degenerative disease of the brainstem (Leigh, 1951, Ebels *et al.*, 1965). It is characterised by symmetrical lesions of the brainstem. Striking biochemical abnormalities associated with this disease are high blood lactate and pyruvate levels (Worsley *et al.*, 1965, Clayton *et al.*, 1967, Hommes *et al.*, 1968, De Groot *et al.*, 1969 Tada *et al.*, 1969a, b) and high plasma alanine levels (Tada *et al.*, 1969a, b). These high blood lactate and pyruvate levels point to an inborn error of carbohydrate metabolism. Post mortem examination of a case studied by Clayton *et al.* (1967) demonstrated a normal conversion of pyruvate into acetyl-CoA and a normal activity of the enzymes lipoate transacetylase, lipoate dehydrogenase, diaphorase, citrate synthase, oxaloacetate carboxylase, fructose-1,6-diphosphatase and phosphofructokinase.

Hommes *et al.* (1968) found in a liver biopsy of a case where the diagnosis was later confirmed by post mortem examination, a normal activity of the enzyme phosphoenolpyruvate carboxykinase but a virtual absence of pyruvate carboxylase, the enzyme which converts pyruvate to oxaloacetate. This observation was confirmed in the case described by Tada *et al.* (1969a, b).

Although these findings support the concept of Leigh's disease being an inborn error of carbohydrate metabolism—and more specifically of gluconeogenesis—its relationship to the neurological damage as observed in this disease is difficult to visualise. Cooper *et al.* (1969) demonstrated that extracts from tissue fluids from a patient suffering from Leigh's disease inhibit thiamine pyrophosphate - adenosine triphosphate phosphotransferase of rat brain mitochondria. They postulate that thiamine triphosphate is the neurophysiologically active form of the vitamin and that in Leigh's disease a factor is present that inhibits the synthesis of thiamine triphosphate.

Therapeutic approaches have consisted of administration of lipoic acid (Clayton *et al.*, 1967, Hommes *et al.*, 1968, De Groot *et al.*, 1969) which causes a fall in the blood lactate and pyruvate level and which seems to have improved the condition of some patients. Lonsdale (1968) was the first to try high doses of thiamine. He claimed an impressive clinical improvement of his patient, who was probably suffering from Leigh's disease. The present communication describes a new case of lactic acidaemia with hyperalaninaemia, from a family unrelated to our earlier studied cases.

Case Report

G. E. was referred to the University Hospital at the age of 14 months. He had a normal birth after an uneventful gestational period of 40 weeks. The birthweight was 3400 g. He was the fifth child in the family, two sisters and two brothers being normal and healthy. The father's father and the mother's mother were first cousins. At the age of 13 months he had chicken pox. Thereafter he developed a clinical picture suggestive of encephalitis. He did not recover completely. He remained somewhat drowsy, but his motor development was apparently unaffected. He could crawl and walk with support at the age of 15 months. At the age of 22 months however he became ataxic. The ataxia worsened periodically and was accompanied by vomiting and hyperpnoea.

Gradually he developed a marked intention tremor.

Routine laboratory investigations showed no abnormalities, except for a high alkaline phosphatase (9·3 Bessey units, normal range 2·8–6·7), which was also present in our earlier cases. There was no generalised aminoaciduria (120 μmoles/kg/24 hrs.). The alanine excretion however was relatively high. Plasma amino acids showed a moderately high alanine level of 0·97 mM (normal range 0·44 $\pm$ 0·20 mM). The other plasma amino acid levels were found to be within normal limits. Acid-base studies revealed a persistent slight metabolic acidosis. Occasionally this acidosis was more pronounced with base deficits of 8-10 meq/l.

Special Investigations

Blood glucose, lactate, pyruvate, β-hydroxybutyrate and acetoacetate were determined enzymatically according to Slein (1965), Hohorst (1965), Bücher *et al.* (1965), Williamson & Mellanby (1965) and Mellanby & Williamson (1965), respectively.

Quantitative amino acid analysis was performed by gradient elution chromatography with a Beckman/Spinco Unichrom amino acid analyser.

Liver pyruvate carboxylase was assayed as described earlier (Hommes *et al.*, 1968), according to Utter & Keech (1963).

Table I summarises some of the results obtained on blood lactate, pyruvate, β-hydroxybutyrate and acetoacetate levels. In the fasting, untreated patient the blood lactate concentration is about five times the normal level. The lactate/pyruvate ratio is however normal. As the blood lactate/pyruvate ratio is an indicator of the intra-cellular, cytoplasmic, redox state (Krebs & Veech, 1970), it can be concluded that no redox reaction is involved in the enzymic defect of Leigh's disease. The same conclusion can be drawn from the β-hydroxy butyrate/

Table I. *Summary of representative levels of blood lactate, pyruvate, β-hydroxybutyrate and acetoacetate of patient G. E. Concentrations are given in mM.*

Patient	*Condition*	*Treatment*	*Lactate*	*Pyruvate*	*Lactate/ pyruvate ratio*	*β-hydroxy- butyrate*	*Aceto- acetate*	*β-hydroxy- butyrate/ acetoacetate ratio*
Control	fasting	none	1·03	0·08	12·9	0·32	0·13	2·50
Control	non-fasting	none	1·35	0·11	12·3	0·046	0·033	1·40
G. E.	fasting	none	4·99	0·39	12·8	0·46	0·21	2·20
G. E.	non-fasting	none	2·30	0·18	12·8	1·07	0·20	5·35
G. E.	fasting	2000 mg thiamine	1·80	0·20	9·1	0·97	0·15	6·40
G. E.	non-fasting	2000 mg thiamine	2·54	0·38	6·7	1·82	0·42	4·32

acetoacetate ratio in the fasting condition, which is an indicator for the redox state of the mitochondrial compartment (Krebs & Veech, 1970).

An alanine loading test according to Fernandes (1971) was then carried out to test alanine as a precursor for glucose. The results are shown in Fig. 1. Despite the high blood alanine level no increase in blood glucose could be observed, suggestive of a defect in gluconeogenesis. This alanine loading test has been carried out under thiamine therapy. It should be noted that both β-hydroxybutyrate and acetoacetate increase (the latter temporarily).

A liver biopsy in which the activity of pyruvate carboxylase was tested confirmed a defect in the gluconeogenic pathway (Table II). Virtually no activity of the enzyme could be detected.

Table II. *Activities of pyruvate carboxylase of rat liver, normal controls and of patient G.E.*
Activities are expressed as μmoles per minute per gram wet weight of tissue.

	Pyruvate carboxylase activity
Adult rat liver	3·0
Control I, aged 14 days	2·1
Control II, aged 1 year	6·2
Patient G.E.	0·14

Administration of lipoic acid resulted only in a slight decrease of blood lactate and pyruvate and no definite clinical improvement was observed. According to Lonsdale (1968) high doses of thiamine were then given. An amount of 2000 mg of thiamine, daily, proved to be effective in lowering the fasting blood lactate and pyruvate levels (Table I). These levels are however still above normal.

During the 5-month period of high thiamine administration the patient had no episodes of ataxia and metabolic acidosis. His clinical condition has improved considerably as has his general performance.

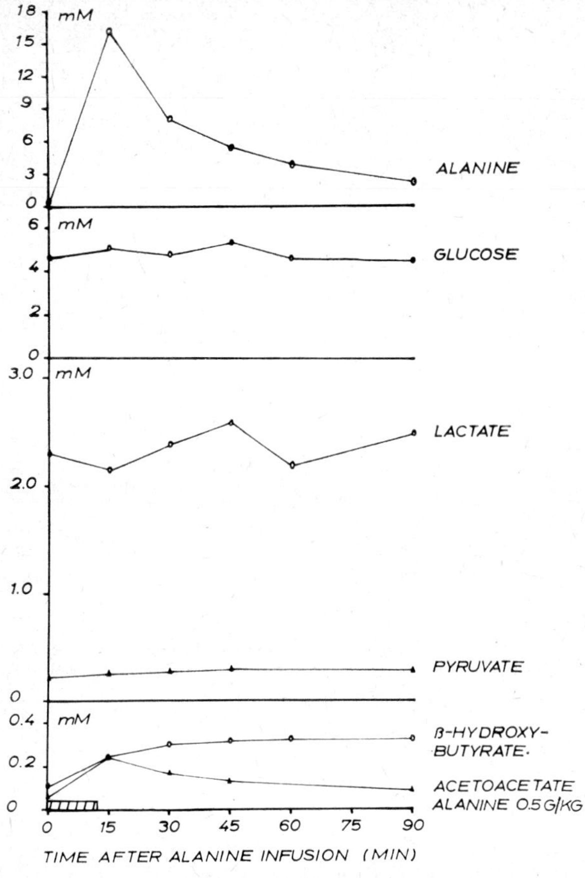

FIG. 1. Concentration of blood alanine, glucose, lactate, pyruvate β-hydroxybutyrate and acetoacetate after alanine loading in patient G.E. Alanine (500 mg/kg bodyweight) was given intravenously in 12 min. Blood samples were taken at the times indicated, deproteinised and analysed.

CONCLUSIONS

The diagnosis of Leigh's encephalomyelopathy is in fact a post mortem diagnosis (Leigh, 1951, Ebels *et al.*, 1965). We can now catalogue three criteria, which characterise this genetically determined disease. First the clinical symptoms, which indicate degeneration of the central nervous system and which manifest themselves at first periodically.

Second, the high blood lactate and pyruvate levels due to a very low activity of pyruvate carboxylase and third, the Wernicke-like autopsy findings.

In the first case described by us (Hommes *et al.*, 1968, De Groot *et al.*, 1969) all three criteria are fulfilled. The case described by Tada *et al.* (1969a, b) reveals two of these criteria, namely the clinical findings and the very low activity of the enzyme pyruvate carboxylase with high blood lactate and pyruvate levels, as does the present case. The third criterion is only evident at post mortem. However, we do know that there are neurological abnormalities suggestive of central nervous system damage, such as absence of tendon reflexes, a marked ataxia and a retardation in motor development. A decrease in blood lactate and pyruvate level by thiamine therapy has been demonstrated in the present study. Previous studies (Clayton *et al.*, 1967, Hommes *et al.*, 1968, De Groot *et al.*, 1969) have shown that administration of lipoic acid also results in a decrease of blood lactate in Leigh's disease. Both lipoic acid and thiamine (as thiamine pyrophosphate) are co-factors of the pyruvate dehydrogenase complex.

An increased activity of this enzyme by the vitamin B_1 treatment would result in an increased production of acetyl-CoA. It can be expected that, due to the deficiency of pyruvate carboxylase, the concentration of oxaloacetate is low. Formation of citrate from acetyl-CoA and oxaloacetate will therefore be low as well. This high acetyl-CoA concentration will result in an increased production of acetoacetate and β-hydroxybutyrate. Indeed, the non-fasting blood levels of β-hydroxybutyrate and acetoacetate were found to be high and even higher during thiamine therapy (Table I), which is consistent with an activation of the pyruvate dehydrogenase complex. These findings do not necessarily contradict a mechanism proposed by Cooper *et al.* (1969) as being responsible for the neurological damage associated with Leigh's disease. Administration of high doses of thiamine seems to be a valuable tool in the treatment of subacute necrotising encephalomyelopathy. Whether this is due to the decreased blood lactate and pyruvate levels observed during thiamine therapy or to a release of the inhibition of the thiamine pyrophosphate-adenosine triphosphate phosphotransferase as suggested by the work of Cooper *et al.* (1969) remains to be established by future research.

The clinical improvement in association with the lower lactate and pyruvate levels on high thiamine therapy suggests that the elevation of lactate and pyruvate and the ensuing metabolic acidosis are directly responsible for at least part of the neurological symptoms.

REFERENCES

Bücher, Th., Czok, R., Lamprecht, W. & Latzko, E. (1965) *In* Bergmeyer, H. U. (ed.), *Methods in Enzymatic Analysis*, p. 253. New York: Academic Press.

Clayton, B. E., Dobbs, R. H. & Patrick, A. D. (1967) *Arch. Dis. Childh.*, **42**, 467.

COOPER, J. R., ITOKAWA, Y. & PINCUS, J. H. (1969) *Science*, **164**, 72.

DE GROOT, C. J., HOMMES, F. A. & JONXIS, J. H. P. (1969) *In Enzymopenic Anaemis, Lysosomes and other Papers, 6th S.S.I.E.M.*, p. 77. Edinburgh: Churchill Livingstone.

EBELS, E. J., BOLKZIJL, E. J. & TROELSTRA, J. A. (1965) *Helv. paediat. Acta*, **20**, 310.

FERNANDES, J. (1971). Personal communication.

HOHORST, H. J. (1965) *In* Bergmeyer, H. U. (ed.), *Methods in Enzymatic Analysis*, p. 266. New York: Academic Press.

HOMMES, F. A., POLMAN, H. A. & REERINK, J. D., (1968) *Arch. Dis. Childh.*, **43**, 423.

KREBS, H. A. & VEECH, R. L. (1970) *In* Sund, H. *Pyridine Nucleotide Dependent Dehydrogenases*, p. 413. Berlin: Springer Verlag.

LEIGH, D. (1951) *J. Neurol. Neurosurg. Psychiat.*, **14**, 216.

LONSDALE, D., (1968) *New Engl. J. Med. 278*, 1235

MELLANBY J. & WILLIAMSON, D. H. (1965) *In Bergmeyer*, H. U. (ed), *Methods in Enzymatic Analysis*, p. 454, New York; Academic Press.

SLEIN, M. W. (1965) *In* Bergmeyer, H. U. (ed.), *Methods in Enzymatic Analysis*, p. 117. New York: Academic Press.

TADA, K., YOSHIDA, T., KONNO, T., WADA, Y. & YOKOYAMA, Y. (1969a), *Tohoku J. exp. Med.*, **97**, 99.

TADA, K., YOSHIDA, T., KONNO, T. & ARAKAWA, T. (1969b), *Tohoku J. exp. Med.*, 99, 121.

UTTER, M. F. & KEECH, D. B. (1963) *J. biol. Chem.*, **238**, 2603.

WILLIAMSON, D. H. & MELLANBY, J. (1965) *In* Bergmeyer, H. U. (ed.), *Methods in Enzymatic Analysis* p. 459. New York: Academic Press.

WORSLEY, H. E., BROOKFIELD, R. E., ELWOOD, J. S., NOBLE, R. L. & TAYLOR, W. H. (1965) *Arch. Dis. Childh.*, **40**, 492.

CONGENITAL LACTIC ACIDOSIS

by

KARL SCHÄRER

HIGH blood lactate levels in early childhood may have various causes, such as prematurity, feeding with acidified milk (Goldmann *et al.*, 1961), dehydration, hypothermia, hypoxia (Greene & Talner, 1964, Huckabee, 1961), primary metabolic disorders (diabetes mellitus, glycogen storage disease), liver disease (Gautier, 1969/70, Perret *et al.*, 1969), sickle cell crisis (Olver, 1969), neoplastic disorders (Field *et al.*, 1966), intoxications, and congenital lactic acidosis (CLA).

Table I. *Reported cases of congenital lactic acidosis. Siblings with a history suggestive of congenital lactic acidosis (not proven by lactate determination) are included, except for the large family reported by Israels* et al. *(1964) and Haworth* et al. *(1967).*
y. = years, mo. = months, d. = days, S. = siblings

Authors	*Age at onset of clinical signs*		*Age at diagnosis*	*Maximal blood lactate mg/100 ml*	*Clinical course*
HARTMANN *et al.*, 1962	1 mo.		4 mo.	209	died at 3½y.
NORDIO *et al.*, 1963, 1967	10 d.		16 d.	103	improved at 7 mo.
ISRAELS *et al.*, 1964	8 mo.		11 mo.	119	died at 2 y.
	3½ mo.		9½ mo.	102	died at 1 y.
ERICKSON, 1965	2 d.	S	3 wk.	254	improved at 7 mo.
	first days	S	17 mo.	205	improved at 20 mo.
WORSLEY *et al.*, 1965	15½ mo.	S	17 mo.	54	died at 2 y.
	3 mo.	S	acidosis: 19 mo.	—	died at 2 y.
HAWORTH *et al.*, 1967	3 mo.	S	3 mo.	162	died at 16 mo.
	1 d.	S	1 d.	61	unchanged at 7 mo.
COHEN *et al.*, 1967	3 mo.		9 mo.	108	improved at 2y.
SCHARER *et al.*, 1968	1 wk.		5 mo.	140	died at 7 mo.
PEYTEL *et al.*, 1969	birth	S		—	died at 8 mo.
	6 wk.	S	10 mo.	42	died at 13 mo.
MARIANI *et al.*, 1970	15 mo.		18 mo.	144	died at 37 mo.
	25 mo.		29 mo.	100	improved at 3 y.
GREENE *et al.*, 1970	first months		8 mo.	165	died at 16½mo.
LIE *et al.*, 1971	3 d.	S	3 d.	—	died at 4 d.
	2 d.	S	3 d.	109	died at 7 d.

CLA is found in a heterogeneous group of patients. The first symptoms are noted between birth and the second year of life. So far sixteen cases have been described in detail (Table I). In addition, three cases were presented in abstract form (Bejar *et al.*, 1968, Brunette *et al.*, 1971). The important *clinical* manifestations of CLA are: periodic attacks of dyspnoea and tachypnoea caused by metabolic acidosis due to the accumulation of l-lactate, pneumonitis, muscular hypotonicity, tetanic signs, generalised convulsions, twitching, tremor, lethargy, which may progress to full coma, psychomotor retardation and, in some patients, obesity, hepatomegaly and cataracts.

The most prominent *biochemical* finding of CLA, metabolic acidosis, may be either transient or constant. During the attacks, the blood pH may fall below 7. The blood ionogram shows an anionic gap. In most patients described so far the lactate concentration in the blood or plasma reached values above 100 mg/100 ml (normal: up to 20 mg/100 ml). The increase in the blood pyruvate levels is less remarkable, thereby often raising the L/P ratio to more than 20. This indicates some degree of tissue hypoxia (Field *et al.*, 1966; Huckabee, 1961 and 1969/70). The high activity of lactic dehydrogenase seems to be a secondary phenomenon. Some patients have been reported with high serum levels of inorganic phosphate, potassium and uric acid (Schärer *et al.*, 1968). Lactate accumulation is also found in the urine and in the cerebrospinal fluid. Occasionally, some other organic acids, such as α-ketoglutarate and amino-acids, were also noted to be raised in urine (Haworth *et al.*, 1967, Schärer *et al.*, 1968, Worsley *et al.*, 1965).

The heterogeneity of CLA can be suspected from the great differences in onset and clinical course. Most patients died during the neonatal period, infancy or early childhood (Table I). A few patients improved, but the follow up period is still too short for a final evaluation of this milder variant of the disease.

In three families siblings were affected, in two other instances the clinical picture of dead siblings was very suggestive of CLA (Peytel *et al.*, 1969, Worsley *et al.*, 1965). The first case described by Israels *et al.* (1964) and the two children reported by Haworth *et al.* (1967) were siblings. In addition to these, five other children in the same family (consisting of a total of twelve siblings) also had attacks of tachypnoea with muscular twitching and coma and died in the first two years of life, without proof of hyperlactataemia.

It appears that from a clinical viewpoint *four types* of CLA can be differentiated at the present time: The first *transitory* type is seen in full-term newborns who *recover* spontaneously in the first months of life (Cohen *et al.*, 1967, Erickson, 1965, Nordio *et al.*, 1963, Nordio & de Pra, 1967). The second type is characterised by an *early fatal course*. Such a case of a full-term newborn who died at 7 days was recently reported from Norway (Lie *et al.*, 1971, Skrede *et al.*, 1971). The third and most prevalent type of CLA comprises children with a *slowly progressive course* starting in the first weeks or months and leading to *death in the first to fourth year* of life (Greene *et al.*, 1970, Hartmann *et al.*, 1962, Haworth *et al.*, 1967, Israels *et al.*, 1964, Peytel *et al.*, 1969, Schärer *et al.*, 1968). In the fourth type, acidotic attacks begin only in the *second year* and usually have a fatal outcome (Mariani *et al.*, 1970, Worsley *et al.*, 1965). This classification of CLA will probably have to be revised as our knowledge of the pathogenesis increases.

It seems that Leigh's *subacute necrotizing encephalomyelopathy*, which is sometimes associated with acidosis (Crome, 1970, Kamoshita *et al.*, 1968) and hyperlactataemia (Clayton *et al.*, 1967, Gruskin *et al.*, 1971, Hommes *et al.*, 1968, Worsley *et al.*, 1965), is difficult to differentiate from CLA, although it usually has a later onset, a more protracted course, is more dominated by neurological manifestations and shows only slight and transient increases of the serum lactate concentration. The anatomical brain lesions observed in both conditions seem to be different (Greene *et al.*, 1970, Peytel *et al.*, 1969, Schärer *et al.*, 1968). Hyperlactataemia has also been found in combination with hyperalaninaemia with psychomotor retardation or intermittent ataxia (Brunette *et al.*, 1971, Lonsdale *et al.*, 1969) and in methylmalonic acidaemia (Oberholzer *et al.*, 1967).

The *treatment* of CLA presents considerable problems as demonstrated by the case presented in Fig. 1. By increasing the dosage of sodium bicarbonate up to 20 g/day the blood pH could be kept within almost normal limits for a long time. The blood lactate ranged between 4 and 16 mmoles/l and had no constant relation to the blood pH nor to the clinical state. The lactate excretion in the urine rose steeply from below 1 g/day to 12 g/day after starting the alkali treatment. The patient showed some improvement in psychomotor development, but died at the age of 7 months from brain oedema and a severe electrolyte imbalance.

The *pathogenesis* of CLA is not clear. However, it seems different from that of idiopathic lactic acidosis in adults (Huckabee, 1961 and 1969/70, Oliva, 1970). It was proposed that in CLA the production of lactate by muscle is increased. Israels *et al.* (1964) found evidence in their case that during exercise the muscles produced increased amounts of lactate. Intravenous loads with lactate and pyruvate showed a decreased metabolism of these organic ions, suggesting failure of the liver's capacity to metabolise lactate by breakdown to CO_2 and gluconeogenesis (Haworth *et al.*, 1967). This would imply a defect in the Cori cycle. In this situation, the kidney has to take over the critical role of removing large amounts of lactate and hydrogen ions (Levy, 1965, Man *et al.*, 1969). The tubular non-ionic diffusion and thereby the renal removal of lactate is facilitated by alkali administration. Lactate accumulation is toxic not only because of the fall in pH, but also through its direct effect, especially on the brain.

Moreover, it appears that lipolysis in adipose tissue is impaired in some patients with CLA, in whom marked obesity and hyperlipidaemia were found (Israels *et al.*, 1964, Schärer *et al.*, 1968). The absence of a rise in the plasma-free fatty acids after injection of a lipolytic agent, human growth hormone, also suggests a blocking of lipid mobilisation. These findings are in good agreement with experimental data which show that lipolysis is reduced by high lactate levels (Bjørntrup, 1965). They also suggest that the function of adipose tissue as an important energy source is impaired in CLA. The lack of free fatty acids and ketone bodies as energy fuels for the working muscle makes the organism more dependent on carbohydrates.

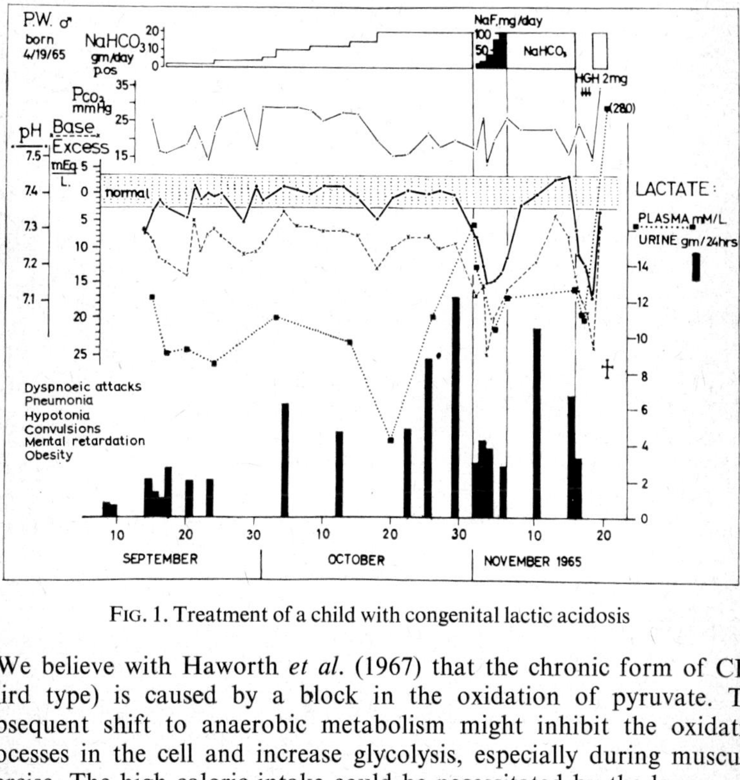

FIG. 1. Treatment of a child with congenital lactic acidosis

We believe with Haworth *et al.* (1967) that the chronic form of CLA (third type) is caused by a block in the oxidation of pyruvate. The subsequent shift to anaerobic metabolism might inhibit the oxidative processes in the cell and increase glycolysis, especially during muscular exercise. The high caloric intake could be necessitated by the low energy yield of anaerobic metabolism. For the latter to continue, a sufficient regeneration of NAD and NADP from their reduced form is required. The progressive course of CLA suggests that a failure occurs in the electron transport chain to re-oxidise NADH, or a defect in the transfer of the extramitochondrial NADH through the mitochondrial membrane. Both mechanisms would explain the deviation from pyruvate to lactate and from triose-phosphate to α-glycerophosphate, thereby increasing lipogenesis. They could also explain the reduced turnover in the Krebs cycle at steps where NAD is needed, e.g. at the step of α-ketoglutarate oxidation. A similar mechanism has recently been suggested in an adult patient with chronic lactic acidosis (Sussmann *et al.*, 1970).

Other pathogenetic mechanisms have to be considered in CLA. In the case of the newborn described by Lie *et al.* (1971) no block in lactate oxidation nor increased glycolysis was found; however, the capacity of the liver to produce glucose was impaired (Skrede *et al.*, 1971). The gluconeogenic pathway was thought to be disturbed in two cases of lactic acidosis with a very different clinical picture (Mariani *et al.*, 1970). The activity of pyruvate carboxylase, a key enzyme of gluconeogenesis, was diminished in the liver of two other children with hyperlactataemia who probably have the same condition (Brunette *et al.*, 1971, Hommes *et al.*, 1968).

REFERENCES

Bejar, R. A., Ando, T., Lopez, P., Cleveland, W. W. & Nyhan, W. L. (1968) *The Society for Pediatric Research*, Atlantic City, NJ., **38**., 158.

Bjørntrup, P. (1965) *Acta med. scand.*, **178**, 253.

Brunette, G. M., Scriver, C. R., Hazel, B. & Delvin, E. (1971) *Int. Congr. Pediat., Vienna*, **5**, 267.

Clayton, B., Dobbs, R. H. & Patrick, A. D. (1967) *Arch. Dis. Childh.*, **42**, 467.

Cohen, A. L., Forgione, H. E. & Dugatkin, S. (1967) *Pren. Med. Argent.*, **54**, 1648.

Crome, L. (1970) *Brain*, **93**, 709.

Erickson, R. J. (1965) *J. Pediat.*, **66**, 1004.

Field, M., Block, J. B., Levin, R. & Rall, D. P. (1966) *Amer. J. Med.*, **40**, 528.

Gautier, E. (1969/70) *Helv. med. Acta*, **35**, 423.

Goldmann, H. I., Karelitz, S., Seifert, E., Acs, H. & Schell, N. (1961) *Pediatrics*, **27**, 921.

Greene, H. L., Schubert, W. K. & Hug, G. (1970) *J. Pediat.*, **76**, 853.

Greene, N. M. & Talner, N. S. (1964) *New Engl. J. Med.*, **270**, 1331.

Gruskin, A. B., Linshaw, M. A., Ettenger, R. B. & Grover, W. (1971) *2nd Sympos. pediat. Nephrol.*, Paris, abstr. p. 103.

Hartmann, A. F., Wohltmann, H., Purkerson, M. L. & Wesley, M. E. (1962) *J. Pediat.*, **61**, 165.

Haworth, J. C., Ford, J. D. & Younoszai, M. K. (1967) *Canad. med. Ass. J.*, **97**, 773.

Hommes, F. A., Polman, H. A. & Reerink, J. D. (1968) *Arch. Dis. Childh.*, **43**, 423.

Huckabee, W. E. (1961) *Amer. J. Med.*, **30**, 833 and 844.

Huckabee, W. E. (1969/70) *Helv. med. Acta*, **35**, 363.

Israels, S., Haworth, J. C., Gourley, B. & Ford, J. D. (1964) *Pediatrics*, **34**, 346.

Kamoshita, S., Aguilar, M. J. & Landing, B. H. (1968) *Amer. J. Dis. Child.*, **116**, 120.

Levy, M. N. (1965) *Proc. N.Y. Acad. Sci.*, **119**, 1029.

Lie, S. O., Löken, A. C., Strömme, J. H. & Aagenaes, Ö. (1971) *Acta paediat. scand.*, **60**, 129.

Lonsdale, D., Faulkner, W. R., Price, J. W. & Smeby, R. S. (1969) *Pediatrics*, **43**, 1025.

Man, N. K., Keller, P., Hallauer, W. & Schirmeister, J. (1969) *Klin. Wschr.*, **47**, 1170.

Mariani, R., Unal, D., Passeron, P., Coignet, J. & Bernard, R. (1970) *Arch. franç. Péd.*, **27**, 617.

NORDIO, S., LAMEDICA, G. M., DE PRA, M. & TROVINI, G. C. (1963) *Minerva pediat.*, **15**, 1068.
NORDIO, S. & DE PRÀ, M. (1967) *Panminerva medica*, **9**, 325.
OBERHOLZER, V. G., LEVIN, B., BURGESS, E. A. & YOUNG, W. F. (1967) *Arch. Dis. Childh.*, **42**, 492.
OLIVA, P. B. (1970) *Amer. J. Med.*, **48**, 209.
OLVER, R. E. (1969) *Proc. Roy. Soc. Med.*, **62**, 1097.
PERRET, A., POLI, S. & ENRICO, F. J. (1969/70) *Helv. med. Acta*, **35**, 377.
PEYTEL, J., SALLE, B., TOMMASI, M., MATHIEU, M., ANTENER, I., ROSENBERG, D. & MONNET, P. (1969) *Arch. franç. Péd.*, **26**, 321.
SCHÄRER, K., MARTY, A. & MUHLETHALER, J. P. (1968) *Helv. paediat. Acta*, **23**, 107.
SKREDE, S., STRÖMME, J. H., STOKKE, O., LIE, S. O. & ELDJARN, L. (1971) *Acta paediat. scand.*, **60**, 138.
SUSSMANN, K. E., ALFREY, A., KIRSCH, W. M. & ZWEIG, P. (1970) *Amer. J. Med.*, **48**, 104.
WORSLEY, H. E., BROOKFIELD, R. W., ELWOOD, J. S., NOBLE, R. L. & TAYLOR, W. H. (1965) *Arch. Dis. Child.*, **40**, 492.

DISCUSSION
(of Papers by Dr de Groot and Dr Schärer)

Watts (*Harrow*). Dr de Groot, did you measure lactate dehydrogenase levels—were the effects of thiamine on lactate levels significant? There were only two pre-treatment points on your table, and one of these lay very close to or within the range of values obtained during treatment.

de Groot (*Groningen*). We measured the lactate dehydrogenase levels in the blood. They were within normal limits. We did not measure the lactate dehydrogenase on the intracellular level. In our table we only have given a few representative values of the pre-treatment levels of lactate and pyruvate. On average, the pre-treatment values were higher than those during treatment.

Sinclair (*London*). I should like to make two points: Firstly, metabolic studies of lactate and pyruvate metabolism have to be undertaken in controlled conditions. The patient must be on a standard diet for at least three days before the tests. Resting values should then be determined followed by the response to a glucose load. Glucose, lactate and pyruvate should be estimated. Dr Levin and I have studied a patient in this way and have found significant changes after the administration of 1000 mg of thiamine per day.

Secondly, I wonder about the significance of changes in the blood lactate when the levels are already high. I feel the changes reported by Drs de Groot and Hommes are difficult to assess because they range from 10–40 times the normal level.

de Groot. It is indeed true that blood lactate and pyruvate should be determined under standard conditions. Next to the diet a standard procedure for the blood sampling is important. Our patient did not receive a true standard diet. The variations in the diet in which these metabolic studies were done, were, however, small and we measured the fasting levels. We did measure glucose levels also. They were within normal limits, and did not alter on thiamine therapy. We are happy to learn that you also have been able to observe a thiamine effect in a patient.

Gompertz (*London*). Three defects in carboxylase activity have been described today involving propionyl CoA, β-methylcrotonyl CoA and pyruvate carboxylase. This is obviously a new group of inborn errors of metabolism. By analogy with the first two carboxylase deficiencies have you tried the effect of biotin?

de Groot. We have, up to 100 mg per day, but without any effect on blood lactate and pyruvate levels, nor on the clinical condition of our patient.

Pollitt (*Sheffield*). Dr de Groot, you have suggested that one of the problems in your patients may be a deficiency of oxaloacetate, interfering in the utilisation of acetyl CoA in the Krebs tricarboxylic acid cycle. Perhaps this would be overcome by feeding aspartate. The extra ammonia available from the transamination would be useful in the correction of acidosis by the kidney and for the synthesis of alanine from pyruvate.

de Groot. This seems a useful suggestion, worthy of detailed study.

Stokke (*Oslo*). Dr de Groot, pyruvate can easily be transaminated to alanine. Where the levels of lactate and pyruvate are high you would also expect the alanine level to be raised. Did you find this?

de Groot. Plasma alanine levels were indeed found to be high (0·72–0·97 mM). As illustrated in Fig. 1 the plasma alanine level with thiamine therapy was considerably lower (0·47 mM).

Baerlocher (*Zurich*). Dr Schärer, I think we should not consider the enzyme pyruvate decarboxylase as the only cause of congenital lactic acidosis. Baker, 1970 (*Lancet*, **2,** 13) reported a patient with fructose-1,6-diphosphatase deficiency who developed lactic acidaemia after a 20-hour fast, and hypoglycaemia after the ingestion of fructose or glycerol. In another report about a patient with the same enzyme defect hyperalaninaemia is also mentioned.

Recently we had the opportunity to study a 14-months old child who presented many of the symptoms of congenital lactic acidosis and who resembled the patient you showed in your film, including the flush*. Lactic acid levels were slightly raised (25–35 mg/100 ml) when the child was in good clinical conditions and on a normal diet. Fructose and glycerol loading produced hypoglycaemia and an increase in lactic acid level to a peak of 78 mg/100 ml. I suggest that your patient, too, may have a deficiency of fructose-1,6-diphosphatase. This defect should be excluded in patients with so-called congenital lactic acidosis.

Schärer (*Heidelberg*). In our patient, hypoglycaemia was never observed. The replacement of sucrose in the diet by galactose did not improve the

* See also *Helv. paediat Acta* **26,** 489, 1971.

clinical state nor decrease the blood lactate and glucose levels. Lactic acidosis was seen during infusion containing glucose as the only carbohydrate. Therefore, I do not believe that our patient had the condition described by Baker and by you, although no acute fructose loading test was performed to exclude this.

Nyhan (*La Jolla*). We have reported in an abstract (*Proc. Soc. pediat. Res.*, 1968, **38**, 158) a patient with lactic acidaemia who also had hyperalaninaemia and some of the clinical manifestations of Leigh's encephalopathy. A liver biopsy specimen was analysed by Dr Huijing in Miami. The activity of pyruvate carboxylase and fructose-1,6-diphosphatase were found to be normal. Abnormal inclusions in the mitochondria were demonstrable with the electron microscope.

de Groot. Not every case with lactic acidaemia and hyperalaninaemia is necessarily due to pyruvate carboxylase deficiency. Any other metabolic pathway of pyruvate utilisation must be considered equally under suspicion and quite a large proportion of pyruvate is oxidised by the mitochondria.

FURTHER STUDIES ON A FAMILY WITH HEPATIC GLYCOGEN SYNTHETASE DEFICIENCY

by

J. RANALD, W. DYKES AND JOHN SPENCER-PEET*

Introduction

Lewis, Spencer-Peet and Stewart (1963) described a family in which mentally retarded identical twins had glucose intolerance, developed hypoglycaemia with convulsions after an overnight fast and gave an adequate blood glucose response following glucagon administered 3 hours after a meal but not in the fasted state. This last finding suggested that the enzymes of glycogenolysis were intact but that there was inability to store glycogen in the liver. This focused attention on the process of formation of glycogen and a liver biopsy carried out on one of the twins revealed normal concentrations of UDPG pyrophosphorylase, phosphorylase and glucose-6-phosphatase, but scanty glycogen and complete absence of activity of the enzyme glycogen synthetase. Histology of the biopsy revealed pronounced fatty change.

The twins' younger sister, Katherine, and older brother, John, exhibited fasting hypoglycaemia, glucose intolerance and showed poor glucose response to glucagon in the fasted state.

At the time of the initial investigation it was not clear why deficiency of glycogen synthetase alone should bring about hypoglycaemia and it was suggested that absence of glycogen in the adrenal cortex in the fasted state might diminish the production of cortisol at a time when it was most needed to stimulate gluconeogenesis. Thus further studies have been carried out on the family (*a*) to see if the ability to prevent fasting hypoglycaemia has improved with time (*b*) to test out the powers of gluconeogenesis and to estimate plasma cortisol concentrations, (*c*) to outline a laboratory test which would be helpful in the differential diagnosis of the condition.

The glucose intolerance in the twins and two of their siblings was attributed to the accumulation of this sugar behind the block in one of its principal pathways of metabolism, viz. its conversion to hepatic glycogen. Since the glucose not utilised for glycogen sythesis must be disposed of in some other way, an overloading of the glycolytic pathway with accumulation of lactic acid might be expected. Hence in this paper an attempt is made to verify this theoretical prediction by following the changes in

* Present address: Department of Chemical Pathology, St Bernard's Hospital, Southall, Middlesex.

blood lactate concentration following the administration of glucose, galactose and glucagon. A comparison is made with the blood lactate values following the administration of these substances in other types of glycogen storage disease as described by Spencer-Peet *et al.* (1971), and also with the changes in blood lactate concentration following the ingestion of galactose in normal children.

Patients

The following members of the family were investigated (Fig. 1):

(*a*) *Dennis*, case 1, and *Stephen*, case 2, born in 1960, the *propositi*,
(*b*) *June*, born in 1956,
(*c*) *John*, born in 1958,
(*d*) *Catherine*, born in 1961.

Six normal children between 10 and 14 years, three male and three female, volunteered as controls for the blood lactate values following oral galactose. The prolonged fast test demonstrated that the twins had some improvement in their ability to prevent hypoglycaemia but glucagon tests performed 3 hours and 20 hours after food gave poor glucose responses, indicating still a poor capacity to store glycogen in the liver. John and Catherine developed frequent bouts of hypoglycaemia during the prolonged fast and the period of carbohydrate-free diet. Their glucagon tests indicated great variability in their capacity to store glycogen, a poor glucose response being obtained 3 hours after food, and a normal one 20 hours after. June is probably normal, since only on a single occasion during the period on a carbohydrate-free diet did she show hypoglycaemia and all her other tests yielded normal results.

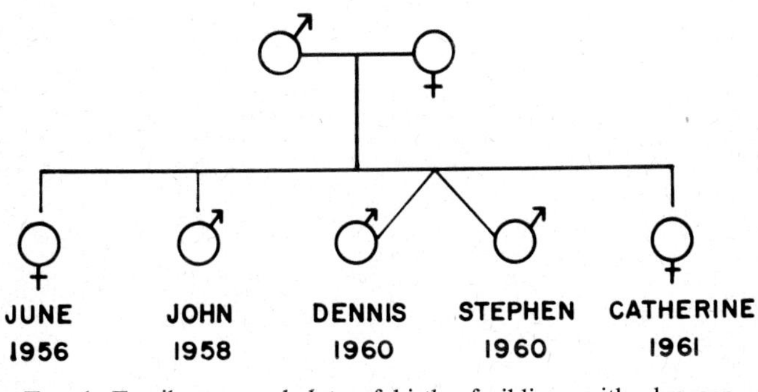

FIG. 1. Family tree and date of birth of siblings with glycogen synthetase deficiency.

In conformity with theoretical prediction the oral glucose and galactose loading tests gave grossly elevated lactate concentrations in John, Catherine, Stephen and Dennis suggesting that the glycolytic pathway was

Table I. *Two hour blood glucose concentrations and blood lactate peaks during oral glucose load test*

Patient	*Year*	*Initial blood glucose (mg/100 ml)*	*2 hour blood glucose (mg/100 ml)*	*Tolerance rating*	*Initial blood lactate (mg/100 ml)*	*Peak blood lactate (mg/100 ml)*
June	1964	113	86	Normal	14·4	16·8
John	1964	43	132	Reduced	14·6	26·4
Stephen (case 2)	1964	49	136	Reduced	9·8	29·0
Dennis (case 1)	1964	57	126	Reduced	10·8	23·2
Catherine	1964	58	131	Reduced	9·7	22·4

Table II. *Blood lactate peak during galactose load test*

Patient	*Year*	*Highest total reducing substance (mg/100 ml)*	*Highest glucose (mg/100 ml)*	*Initial blood lactate (mg/100 ml)*	*Blood lactate peak (mg/100 ml)*
June	1964	118	73	11·8	16·8
John	1964	213	121	15·3	37·8
	1969	150	105	10·5	63·0
Stephen	1964	167	118	12·0	36·2
(case 2)	1969	190	147	13·8	66·0
Dennis	1964	131	111	10·1	32·5
(case 1)	1969	165	135	9·5	55·0
Catherine	1964	154	120	14·2	34·0
	1969	173	153	14·9	53·0

Table III. *Differential diagnosis of glycogen storage disease by various tests*

Hepatic enzyme defect	*Fasting hypoglycaemia*	*Oral galactose load*		*Fasting glucagon test*	
		Blood glucose	*Blood lactate*	*Blood glucose*	*Blood lactate*
Glucose-6-phosphatase (very large liver)	Severe	No rise	Marked rise	No rise	Marked rise
Amylo 1–6 glucosidase	Moderate or severe	Rise	No rise	No rise fasted (small rise after meal)	No rise
Phosphorylase	Mild or moderate	Rise	No rise	No rise fasted (small rise when fed well)	No rise
Glycogen synthetase (no liver enlargement)	Severe	Rise	Marked rise	No rise fasted (small rise when fed well)	No rise
Normal child	Nil	Rise	No rise	Brisk rise	No rise

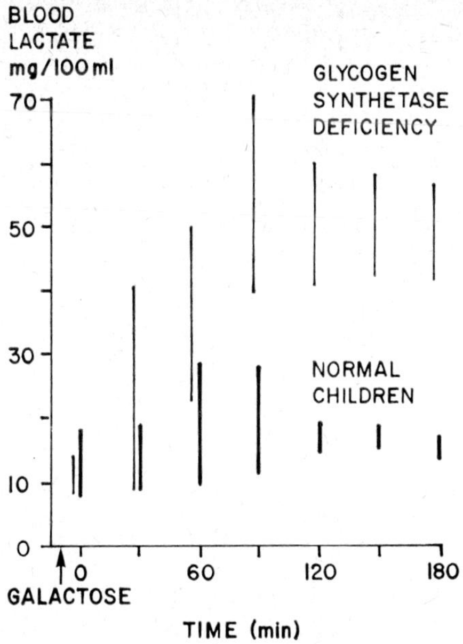

FIG. 2. The range of blood lactate concentrations following oral galactose in normal children and in children with glycogen synthetase deficiency.

being used as an alternative to glycogen storage (Tables I and II and Fig. 2). As further confirmation of the theoretical prediction one would anticipate higher concentrations of blood glucose following galactose in the children with this lesion than in normal children, and as can be seen in Fig. 3 this is indeed the case. However, there is no obvious explanation for the larger overproduction of lactate after galactose as compared to glucose in the four children with the disease (Fig. 4). The absence of elevation in the blood lactate concentration following administration of glucagon further suggests that there is scanty glycogen in the liver to produce glucose and thence lactate.

Measurement of blood lactate concentrations following administration of glucose, galactose and glucagon have been used in the differential diagnosis of various forms of hepatic glycogen storage disease (Fernandes, Huijing & Van de Kamer, 1969; Spencer-Peet *et al.*, 1971). This latter study has shown that deficiency of hepatic glycogen synthetase gives a pattern of results in these tests which is different from those found in other hypoglycaemic conditions associated with deficiencies of enzymes involved in hepatic glycogen metabolism (Table III). However significant numbers from the series of children with evidence of hepatic glycogen

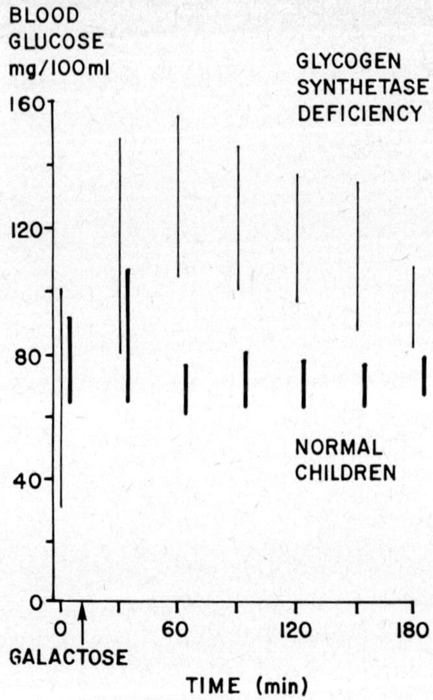

FIG. 3. The range of blood glucose concentrations following galactose in normal children and children with glycogen synthetase deficiency.

storage disease reported by Spencer-Peet *et al.* (1971), while giving patterns typical of a particular enzyme defect, were found to have normal amounts of this enzyme when the latter was assayed in a liver biopsy. Hence, certainty of diagnosis must still depend on the satisfactory demonstration of an enzyme deficiency in such material. None the less, results from these simple tests with galactose, glucose and glucagon will continue to give valuable information in the early stages of investigation and diagnosis of inborn errors of hepatic glycogen metabolism.

Another approach to this problem of definitive diagnosis is the estimation of glycogen synthetase concentrations in red or white blood cells. Normal quantities of this enzyme were found in the former cells by Spencer-Peet (1964). Preliminary assays on white blood cells have yielded conflicting results (Toothill & Ridley, 1971).

Another question to be asked is whether this family is unique in the world literature. One other case described by Parr *et al.* (1965) died within a few months of birth, had hepatomegaly and complete absence of

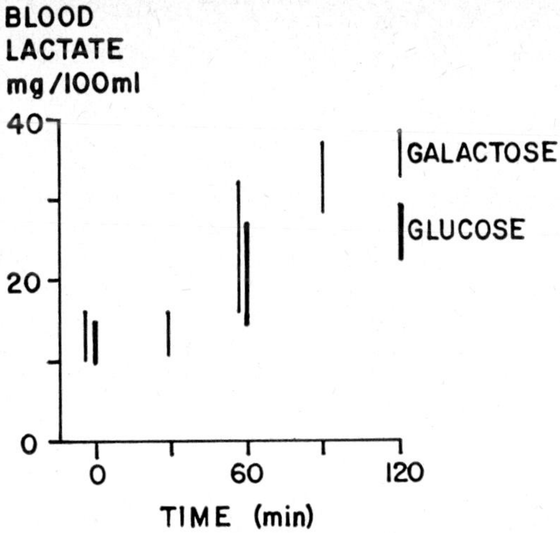

FIG. 4. Range of blood lactate concentrations after glucose and galactose in children with glycogen synthetase deficiency.

glycogen from liver, muscles and adrenal cortices and absent activity of both glycogen synthetase and phosphorylase in liver and skeletal muscles. Both our own case, Dennis, and Parr's case had fatty change in the liver. Some of the features of our case are different from those of Parr *et al.* (1965); the former was not diagnosed until the age of 15 months; he had no hepatomegaly and there was some glycogen present in the liver biopsy and normal activity of phosphorylase. However, in the case reported by Parr *et al.* (1965) investigations were done on autopsy material which may have accounted for the absence of glycogen and phosphorylase. On balance, however, it would seem that the two cases are not identical.

SUMMARY

As follow-up studies on a family with hepatic glycogen synthetase deficiency, the blood glucose concentrations were measured during glucagon tests, and both blood glucose and plasma cortisol were determined during periods of prolonged fasting and isocaloric carbohydrate-free diets. The twins on whom the original diagnosis was made are now better able to maintain their blood glucose level and prevent hypoglycaemia, but their ability to store glycogen inthe liver is still extremely poor.

John, the twins' elder brother, and Catherine, their younger sister, still have frequent episodes of hypoglycaemia, still have a diminished capacity to convert glucose to glycogen, and their ability to store glycogen in the liver is variable. June, the twins' elder sister, is normal. Measurement of blood lactate concentrations after oral administration of glucose, and more particularly galactose, is a useful test in the differential diagnosis of hepatic glycogen synthetase deficiency. However, for definitive diagnosis of the condition a liver biopsy with assay of individual enzymes is still essential.

REFERENCES

Fernandes, J., Huijing, F. & Van de Kamer, J. H. (1969) *Arch. Dis. Childh*, **44**, 311.

Lewis, G. M., Spencer-Peet, J. & Stewart, K. M. (1963) *Arch. Dis. Childh.*, **38**, 40.

Spencer-Peet, J., Norman, M. E., Lake, B. D., McNamara, J. & Patrick, A. D. (1971) *Quart. J. Med.*, **40**, 95.

Spencer-Peet, J. (1964) *Clin. chim. Acta*, **10**, 481.

Parr, J., Teree, T. M. & Larner, J. (1965) *Pediatrics*, **35**, 770.

Toothill, C. & Ridley, J. (1971) Personal communication.

DISCUSSION
(of the Paper by Dr Dykes)

Harris (*Sheffield*). Was the catecholamine output measured?

Dykes (*Leeds*). The urinary 24-hours catecholamine output was measured on several occasions, in each child and in each case the values were normal.

Watts (*Harrow*). What was the activity of glycogen synthetase in leucocytes, fibroblasts or other tissues?

Dykes. There were normal concentrations of glycogen synthetase in erythrocytes (Spencer-Peet, 1964). The preliminary investigations of the level of the enzyme in leucocytes have given contradictory results (Toothill, 1971, personal communication). No other tissues have been looked at for enzyme assays.

Sinclair (*London*). Was muscle glycogen looked at and were adrenaline tests done?

Dykes. Adrenaline tests were done on the twins in 1962 and there was a satisfactory rise of blood sugar after administration subcutaneously of adrenalin following an overnight fast (case 1, 40 mg; case 2, 50 mg). This was interpreted as being due to the breakdown of muscle glycogen but no direct measurements of muscle glycogen synthetase have ever been made. Since 1962 the glucagon test has been used as a more critical index of liver glycogen storage.

Crawfurd (*Leeds*). Have you investigated the parents with a galactose load or other tests? Would you comment on the possibility that John and Catherine may be heterozygotes rather than homozygotes?

Dykes. The mother gave a normal glucose tolerance test. The father was investigated for glycosuria when 8 years of age and gave a lag type of glucose tolerance curve. Neither of the parents would allow any further tests to be carried out on them. It is very possible that John and Catherine are heterozygous for the condition and the twins are homozygous for the condition. However, the determination of this will depend on the discovery of an alternative method to liver biopsy to demonstrate deficiency of glycogen synthetase.

Bickel (Heidelberg). In an early case of von Gierke's disease I was struck by the fact that the patient did not develop brain damage although for several years he had repeated and prolonged periods of hypoglycaemia. It is remarkable that there is not a close correlation between hypoglycaemia and brain damage in such cases. Some of your patients showed pronounced hypoglycaemia. Were they mentally retarded?

Dykes. The twins on whom the original diagnosis was made are mentally retarded. The other members of the family are of normal mental development.

p-HYDROXYPHENYLPYRUVIC ACID METABOLISM IN HEREDITARY TYROSINAEMIA

Abstract of Paper by

B. N. La Du

Patients with hereditary tyrosinaemia show a consistent reduction in liver p-hydroxyphenylpyruvic acid (pHPPA) oxidase activity, liver cirrhosis, and defective renal reabsorption of amino acids, glucose and phosphate. The hypertyrosinaemia and tyrosyluria associated with the liver and kidney abnormalities in these patients have led to the suggestion that a hereditary deficiency of pHPPA oxidase accounts for the biochemical and clinical features of the disorder. Enzymatic studies in our laboratory with liver obtained at autopsy and biopsy from over twenty-five patients with tyrosinaemia show a marked reduction, but not a complete loss, of pHPPA oxidase activity. Tyrosine transaminase and phenylalanine hydroxylase are also significantly reduced. Nevertheless, it is probable that altered tyrosine metabolism in this hereditary disease is secondary to another metabolic defect, as yet unknown, which results in inhibition of pHPPA oxidase. The accumulation of tyrosine metabolites, pHPPA and its metabolic derivatives, seems to contribute to the renal and liver damage since dietary restriction of tyrosine intake ameliorates the metabolic disease. Some of the alternative pathways of pHPPA metabolism include reduction to p-hydroxyphenyllactic acid by aromatic ketoacid reductase, and conversion of pHPPA to p-hydroxy phenylbenzaldehyde and p-hydroxybenzoic acid by oxidative cleavage of the side chain. Possible mechanisms by which the formation of these metabolites could contribute to the liver and kidney damage will be presented. Why tyrosyl metabolites can be toxic in hereditary tyrosinaemia but not in other conditions of altered tyrosine metabolism (such as vitamin C deficiency and premature infants with tyrosyluria) will be discussed.

METABOLISM OF p-HYDROXYPHENYLPYRUVATE IN HEREDITARY TYROSINAEMIA

by

BENGT LINDBLAD, GÖRAN LINDSTEDT, SVEN LINDSTEDT AND MARIANNE RUNDGREN

Catecholamines and δ-Aminolaevulinic Acid in Hereditary Tyrosinaemia

IN the course of the last 5 years we have had the opportunity to study ten cases of hereditary tyrosinaemia, which have all presented the characteristic signs and symptoms of the disease (Bodegård *et al.*, 1969; Gentz *et al.*, 1965; Gentz *et al.*, 1967).* Apart from these findings we have also noted some other biochemical abnormalities in the disease. One patient (a 14-year-old girl, M.S.) had episodes of arterial hypertension and was found to have a very high urinary excretion of catecholamines and an increased excretion of 4-hydroxy-3-methoxymandelic acid (Fig. 1) (Gentz *et al.*, 1970). As seen from Table I a high excretion of catecholamines was

Table I. *Urinary excretion of epinephrine, norepinephrine, 4-hydroxy-3-methoxymandelic acid and δ-aminolaevulinic acid in 7 cases with hereditary tyrosinaemia*

Patient	*Age years*	*Epinephrine µg/day*	*Norepinephrine µg/day*	*4-Hydroxy-3-methoxy mandelic acid mg/day*	*δ-Amino-laevulinic acid mg/g creatinine*
P.W.	2/12	0·8–1	1– 3	—	71–104
R.M.	1	1–6	5–44	—	50–250
A.W.	5	2–45	6·5–59	0·2–3·2	9–16
M.F.	11	3·5–4	8–16	—	28–53
M.S.	15	6–90	19–329	0–29	80–250
E.E.	17	—	—	—	49–62
K.J.	17	2–14	11–43	4·9—27	46–60
Normal adults		<15	<50	<7	<5

then found to be common in patients with hereditary tyrosinaemia. The same patient as well as another (a 4-year-old boy, A.W.) on several occasions had crises with abdominal pains and peripheral pareses, resembling the crises seen in acute porphyria, which caused us to measure the excretion of δ-aminolaevulinic acid. In these two cases, as well as in all our other patients, the excretion of δ-aminolaevulinic acid was increased (Table I) (Gentz *et al.*, 1969b). This therefore is a sign which is as

* Most of these patients have been under the care of Professor Rolf Zetterström and Dr Johan Gentz at the Department of Pediatrics, St Göran's Hospital, Karolinska Institute, Stockholm.

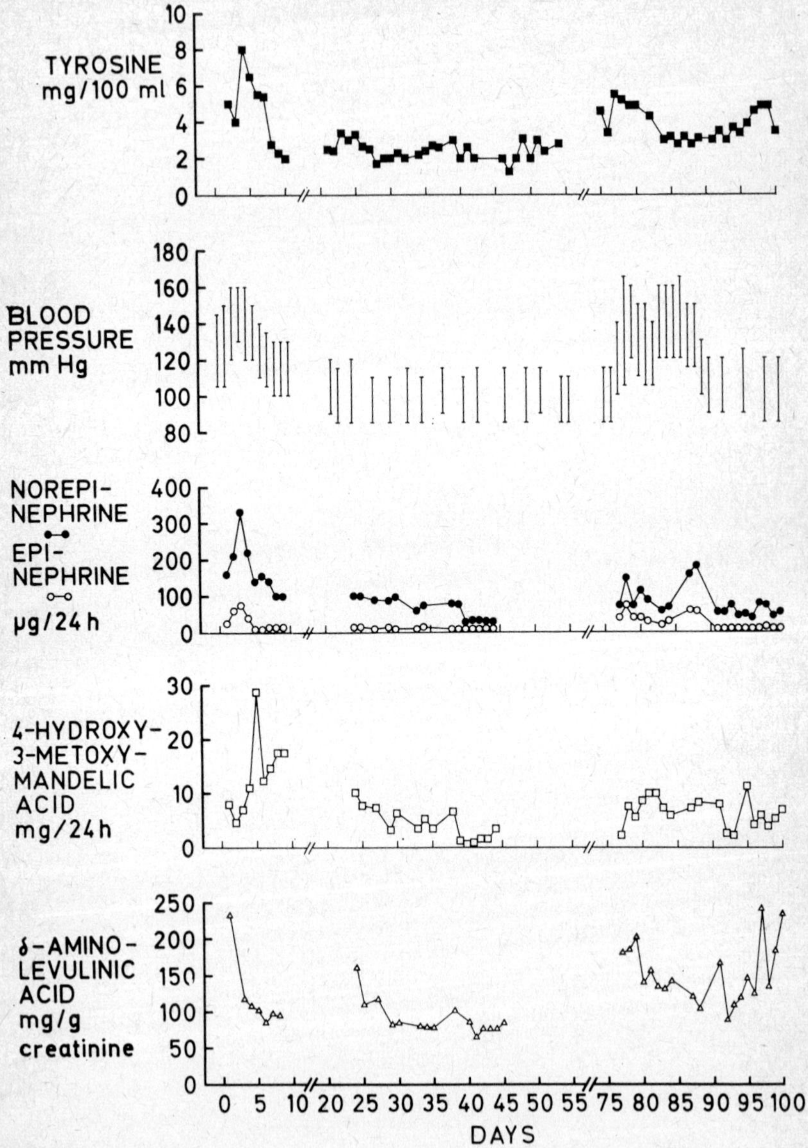

FIG. 1. Serum tyrosine concentration, systolic and diastolic blood pressures and the urinary excretion of norepinephrine, epinephrine, 4-hydroxy-3-methoxymandelic acid and δ-aminolaevulinic acid during two hypertensive crises in a 14-year-old girl (M.S.) with hereditary tyrosinaemia.

characteristic of the disease as the high tyrosine concentration in plasma and the high urinary excretion of phenolic acids. At present we can suggest no biochemical link between the altered tyrosine metabolism and the increased excretion of a porphyrin precursor. Interestingly, we have in several patients observed an increase in the excretion of δ-aminolaevulinic acid during loading with p-hydroxyphenylpyruvate or with phenylalanine (Gentz *et al.*, 1971). It is well known that δ-aminolaevulinic acid synthetase activity may be induced by several aromatic compounds but none of those normally occuring in the degradation of tyrosine has been reported to act in this way. It may be of interest that we have found a high activity of δ-aminolaevulinic acid synthetase in a hepatoma removed from the 14-year-old girl mentioned above (Gentz *et al.*, 1969a) and that Kang and Gerald (1970) have recently reported similar results with liver tissue from their case. The fact that the excretion of porphobilinogen is not elevated indicates that the primary cause of the high excretion of δ-aminolaevulinic acid is an inhibition of δ-aminolaevulinic acid dehydratase (EC 4.2.1.24).

Plasma Concentration and Urinary Excretion of p-Hydroxyphenylpyruvate

The first steps in the degradation of tyrosine are: (i) transamination to p-hydroxyphenylpyruvate catalysed by tyrosine aminotransferase (EC 2.6.1.5), and (ii) conversion of p-hydroxyphenylpyruvate to homogentisate catalysed by p-hydroxyphenylpyruvate hydroxylase (EC 1.14.2.2). Recently Fellman *et al.* (1969) have described a case in which a deficiency of cytoplasmic tyrosine aminotransferase is believed to be the reason for the elevated plasma tyrosine concentration. The other cases in which biochemical studies have been carried out all appear to have a defect in the degradation of p-hydroxyphenylpyruvate. The serum concentration of p-hydroxyphenylpyruvate is increased above normal in hereditary tyrosin-

Table II. *Serum concentrations of tyrosine and p-hydroxyphenylpyruvate in five cases of hereditary tyrosinaemia. The p-hydroxyphenylpyruvate concentration was determined by a modification of the enol-borate method* (*Gentz* et al., *1969c*) *and tyrosine according to Waalkes and Udenfriend* (*1957*)

Patient	*Tyrosine*	*p-Hydroxyphenylpyruvate* (*mg/100 ml*)
K.J.	6·7–10·3	0·31–0·39
M.S.	2·4–6·7	0·07–0·12
M.F.	4·0	0·11
A.W.	3·3	0·09
P.W.	2·7	0·07
Normal controls	1·6–2·3	$<0{\cdot}05$

aemia (Table II) (Gentz *et al.*, 1969c). It must be assumed that the relation between the concentration of tyrosine and p-hydroxyphenylpyruvate is to a large extent determined by the equilibrium in the reaction catalysed by the tyrosine aminotransferases. The present data indicate that the increase in p-hydroxyphenylpyruvate concentration above normal is sufficient to explain the high plasma tyrosine concentration. p-Hydroxyphenylpyruvate is rapidly eliminated from the blood (Fig. 2) and has a high renal clearance (Table III). By a gas-

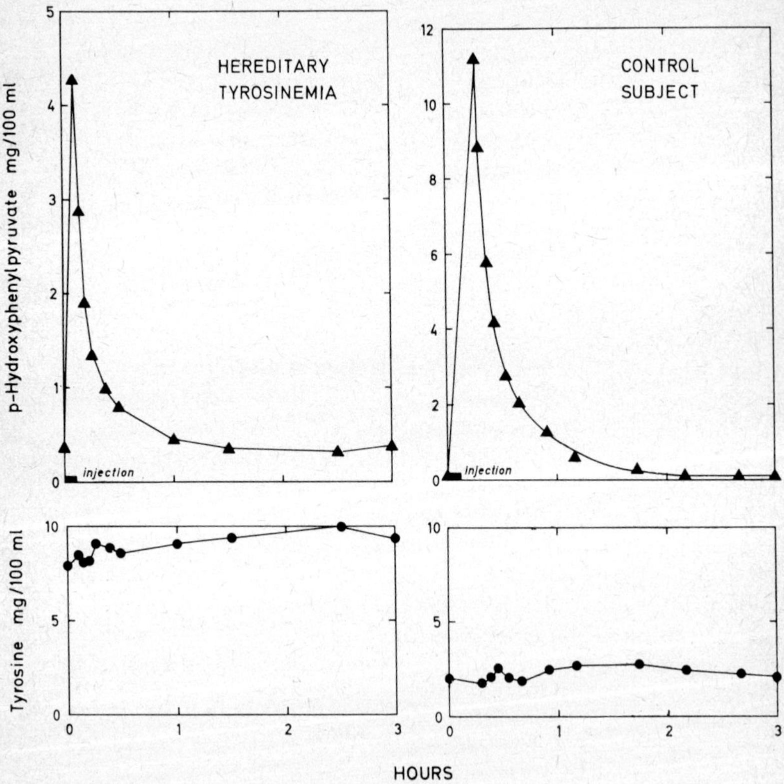

FIG. 2. Elimination of p-hydroxyphenylpyruvate from plasma in a patient with hereditary tyrosinaemia (*left*) and in a control subject (*right*). The lower part shows the plasma tyrosine concentration. The subjects received 13 mg/kg and 40 mg/kg body weight of sodium p-hydroxyphenylpyruvate by intravenous injection during the time indicated in the figure. The p-hydroxyphenylpyruvate concentration was determined by a modification of the enol-borate method (Gentz *et al.*, 1969c) and tyrosine according to Waalkes and Udenfriend (1957).

chromatographic method the phenolic acids in urine have been quantitated after injection of p-hydroxyphenylpyruvate. In the patients studied 90-110 per cent of the injected amount has been accounted for in the urine, whereas in normal subjects about 30 per cent of an intravenous load is recovered in the urine (Gentz *et al.*, 1969c).

Table III. *Renal clearance of p-hydroxyphenylpyruvate in three cases of hereditary tyrosinaemia. p-Hydroxyphenylpyruvate in plasma and urine was determined with an enol-borate method and with gas-liquid chromatography, respectively, on samples obtained during oral* L*-phenylalanine tolerance tests* (*Gentz* et al., *1969c*)

Case	*Renal clearance of p-hydroxyphenylpyruvate, ml/min/1·73 m²*
M.F.	547
K.J.	558
R.M.	488

Determination of p-Hydroxyphenylpyruvate Hydroxylase Activity in Fine-Needle Biopsies

It is apparent from published data that in some cases of hereditary tyrosinaemia there is no detectable enzyme activity in the liver, whereas in other cases a significant activity is found (Gentz *et al.*, 1965; La Du, 1967; These determinations have been performed on autopsy material or on wedge biopsies obtained at surgery. We have considered it of interest to develop a method which would make it possible to make repeat determinations in one and the same patient in order to follow the course of the disease and the effect of dietary treatment (Lindblad, 1971). The present method involves measurement of the enzyme product, i.e. homogentisate, and there is thus no interference by degradation of p-hydroxyphenylpyruvate to other products like p-hydroxyphenylacetate. The steps in the procedure are listed in Table IV and the composition of the incubation mixture is given in Table V. Fig. 3 shows the results obtained in a control case, in a case of hereditary tyrosinaemia with less

Table IV. *Steps in the determination of p-hydroxyphenylpyruvate hydroxylase activity in fine-needle aspiration biopsies of human liver*

1. Preparation of *p*-hydroxy[U–^{14}C]phenylpyruvate from L-[U–^{14}C]tyrosine with L-amino acid oxidase.
2. Homogenization of liver biopsy.
3. Centrifugation at 40,000 x g.
4. Incubation of supernatant (See Table V).
5. Thin-layer chromatography.
6. Scanning of thin-layer plate for isotope distribution (see Fig. 3).

Table V. *Composition of the incubation mixture in the assay of p-hydroxyphenylpyruvate hydroxylase activity*

1. Enzyme, 40,000 x g supernatant	0·1–0·5	mg liver
2. Catalase	1·6	mg/ml
3. Reduced 2,6-dichlorophenolindophenol	0·15	mM
4. Reduced glutathione	10	mM
5. 2,2′-Dipyridyl	1·0	mM
6. p-Hydroxy[U-^{14}C]phenylpyruvate	0·1	mM
7. Potassium phosphate buffer, pH 6·5	100	mM

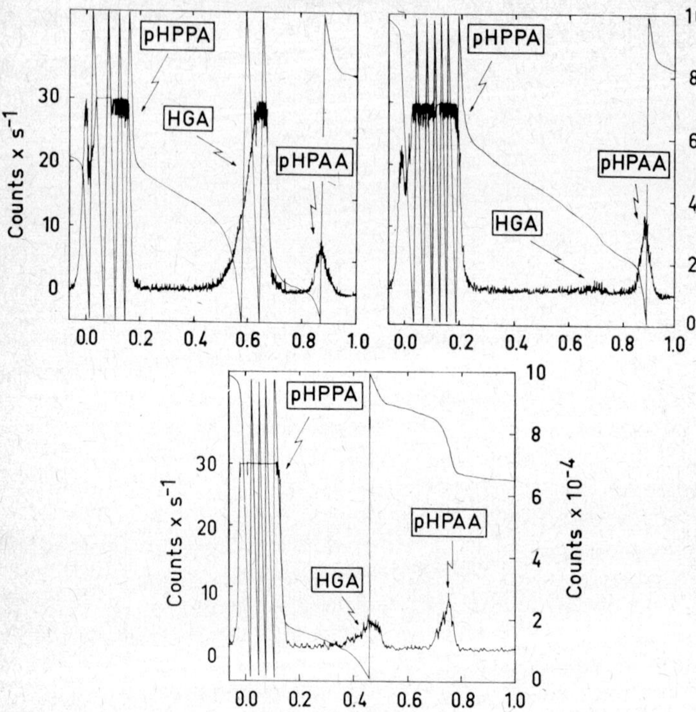

FIG. 3. Determination of p-hydroxyphenylpyruvate hydroxylase activity in fine-needle aspiration liver biopsies from control subject (*left*), patient with hereditary tyrosinaemia with less than 1 per cent of control activity (*right*) and patient with residual activity (*lower*). The procedure given in Table IV was followed. The figure shows the final scan for isotope distribution on the TLC-plates. The recording was made with a Berthold thin layer scanner equipped with an integrator.

than 1 per cent of control enzymic activity, and in another case with significant residual activity of p-hydroxyphenylpyruvate hydroxylase.

Since p-hydroxyphenylpyruvate hydroxylase is a soluble enzyme the tissue fragments obtained by fine-needle biopsy cannot be washed free of admixed blood without loss of enzyme, and the enzyme activity can therefore not be expressed relative to tissue weight or to protein content in the biopsy. We have chosen to relate the enzyme activity to the activity of a number of other cytoplasmic liver enzymes (Table VI) which have been determined with microfluorometric techniques in the same biopsy (Gentz and Lindblad, 1971). Fig. 4 shows the variation in results which is obtained when duplicate biopsies are performed on the same patient. If the activity of p-hydroxyphenylpyruvate hydroxylase is expressed relative

Table VI. *Cytoplasmic liver enzymes used as reference in the determination of p-hydroxyphenylpyruvate hydroxylase activity in fine-needle aspiration biopsies of human liver*

Alanine aminotransferase (EC 2.6.1.2) GPT
Aspartate aminotransferase (EC 2.6.1.1) GOT
Glycerol-3-phosphate dehydrogenase (EC 1.1.1.8) GDH
Lactate dehydrogenase (EC 1.1.1.27) LDH
Sorbitol dehydrogenase (EC 1.1.1.14) SDH

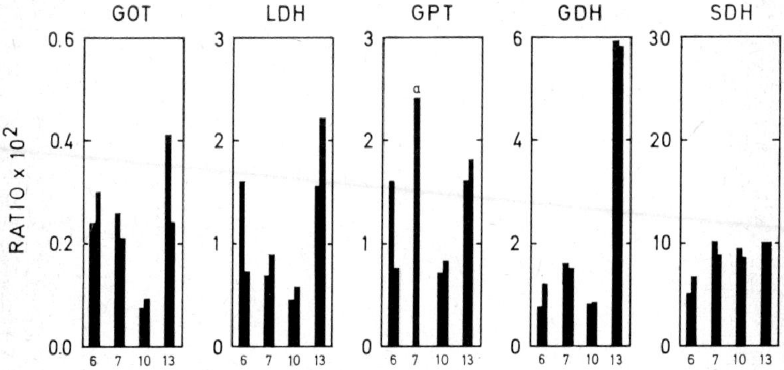

FIG. 4. Determination of p-hydroxyphenylpyruvate hydroxylase activity in duplicate fine-needle aspiration liver biopsies. In each subject two biopsies were obtained on the same occasion. Enough material was not left for analysis of GPT in the second biopsy in subject 7(a). The enzyme activity has been related to that of five reference enzymes (see Table VI).

to the reference enzymes there is no significant difference between subjects without known liver disease and a group of patients with liver cell damage (Fig. 5). Fig. 5 also shows the results from biopsies performed in four cases of hereditary tyrosinaemia. In two of these cases (no. 1, M.F. and no. 4, R.M.) significant enzyme activity could be detected (1 and 9 per cent controls). In the other two cases (no. 2, Ka.J. and no. 3, K.J.) no enzyme activity was recorded but on the basis of the sensitivity of the method it can be stated that in these two subjects the enzyme activity could not have been more than 11 and 1 per cent of the control values. Included in Fig. 5 is the result from a determination of the enzyme activity in a liver biopsy obtained from the mother of two affected children. The enzyme activity fell within the range of the controls in this subject, heterozygous for the disease.

Properties of p-Hydroxyphenylpyruvate Hydroxylase from Human Liver

The enzyme p-hydroxyphenylpyruvate hydroxylase has been partially purified from animal sources (Hager *et al.*, 1957; Taniguchi *et al.*, 1964). It has some interesting properties, e.g. a stimulation by catalase and a

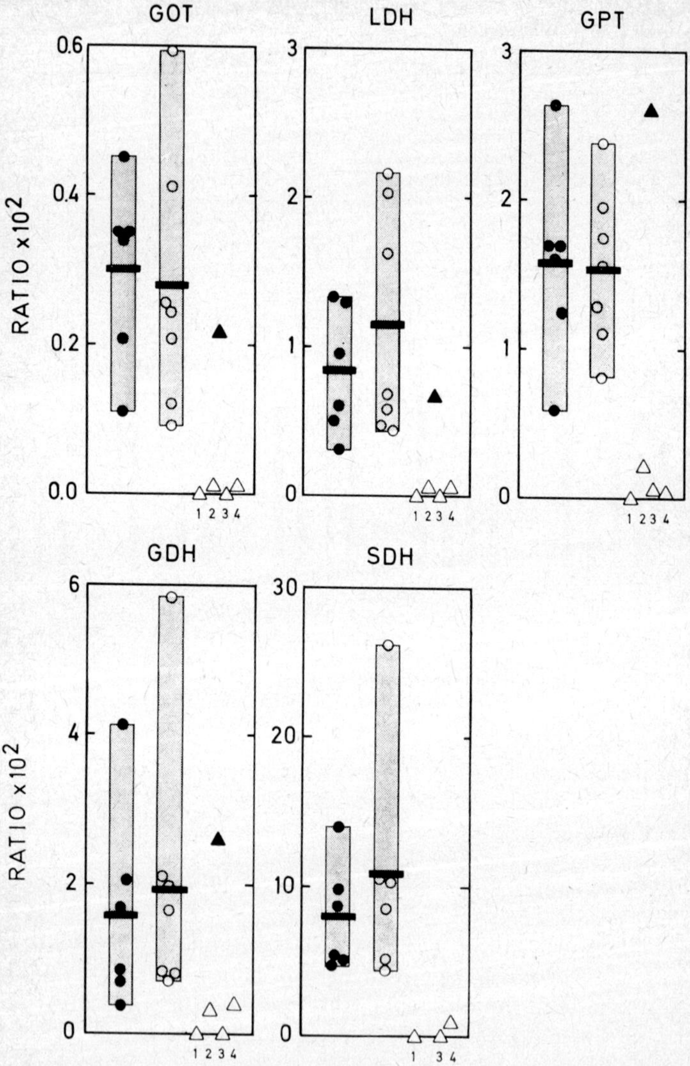

FIG. 5. ● = Ratio between p-hydroxyphenylpyruvate hydroxylase activity and the activity of GOT, LDH, GPT, GDH and SDH in reference subjects without liver disease ○ = reference subjects with liver disease ▲ = one heterozygote for hereditary tyrosinaemia △ = four patients with hereditary tyrosinaemia. The bar represents the mean value and the dashed area the range.

marked reaction inhibition, particularly in the absence of reducing agents like dichlorophenolindophenol or ascorbate (Zannoni & La Du, 1956, 1959). The possibility has been discussed that low activity of p-hydroxyphenylpyruvate hydroxylase in hereditary tyrosinaemia is due to the formation of an enzyme inhibitor or to a condition in the liver which inactivates the enzyme. To examine such hypotheses a more detailed knowledge of the human enzyme is needed. We have now purified the human enzyme by a series of chromatographic procedures and can report on some properties of the enzyme. By chromatography on TEAE-cellulose it was possible to separate the enzyme activity into three fractions which correspond to three protein bands on agarose-gel electrophoresis (Fig. 6).

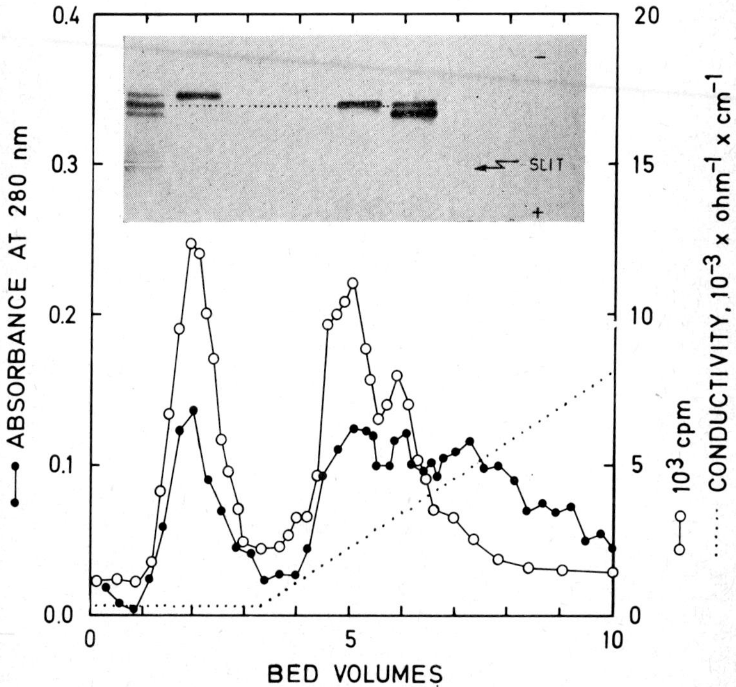

FIG. 6. TEAE-cellulose chromatography of partially purified p-hydroxy-phenylpyruvate hydroxylase from human liver. Protein (110 mg) was applied to a column (2·5 × 20 cm) of Serva TEAE-cellulose equilibrated with 5 mM TRIS-HCl buffer, pH 7·9. Elution was started with two bed volumes of this buffer followed by a linear KCl-gradient (0-150 mM KCl) in 5 mM TRIS-HCl buffer. Protein, ● —— ●; p-hydroxyphenyl-pyruvate hydroxylase activity ○ —— ○. Inserted is the result of agarose gel electrophoresis (1 per cent agarose, 0·5 M pyridinium chloride buffer at pH 6·3) of the material applied to the column (*left*) and of material from the respective peaks.

By a slightly different procedure we have obtained a preparation of the enzyme which gave a single peak when chromatographed on a column of Sephadex G-200 (Lindblad *et al.*, 1971). Ultracentrifugation with the sedimentation equilibrium method (Yphantis, 1964) indicated a molecular weight of 90–100,000 in good agreement with the gel-chromatography data shown in Fig. 7. This preparation contained less than 0·02 mole of

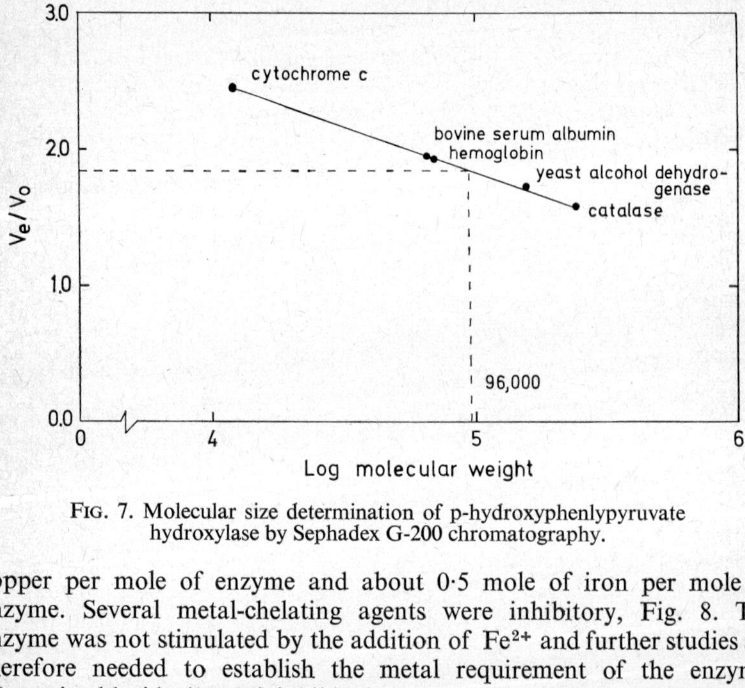

FIG. 7. Molecular size determination of p-hydroxyphenlypyruvate hydroxylase by Sephadex G-200 chromatography.

copper per mole of enzyme and about 0·5 mole of iron per mole of enzyme. Several metal-chelating agents were inhibitory, Fig. 8. The enzyme was not stimulated by the addition of Fe^{2+} and further studies are therefore needed to establish the metal requirement of the enzyme. Mercuric chloride (1 mM) inhibited the enzyme to 45 per cent but other SH-reagents (e.g. o-iodosobenzoate, iodoacetate, ethylmaleimide, and arsenite) caused no inhibition at the same concentration. Table VII shows

Table VII. *p-Hydroxyphenylpyruvate and phenylpyruvate as substrates for human p-hydroxyphenylpyruvate hydroxylase*

	p-Hydroxyphenylpyruvate keto $U x g^{-1}$	enol $U x g^{-1}$	*Phenylpyruvate* keto $U x g^{-1}$	*Ratio*
Acetone powder extract	7·2	—	0·094	77
Purified enzyme	857	<8	12·9	68

that the ratio between the enzyme activities measured with phenyl-pyruvate and p-hydroxyphenylpyruvate as substrate remained constant

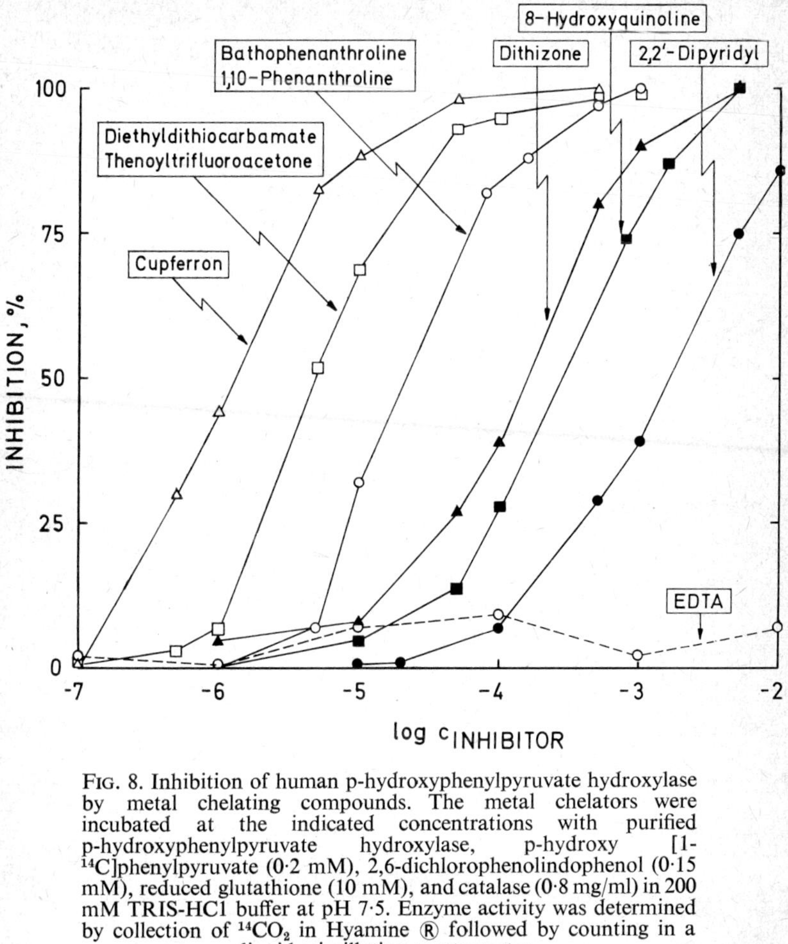

FIG. 8. Inhibition of human p-hydroxyphenylpyruvate hydroxylase by metal chelating compounds. The metal chelators were incubated at the indicated concentrations with purified p-hydroxyphenylpyruvate hydroxylase, p-hydroxy [1-^{14}C]phenylpyruvate (0·2 mM), 2,6-dichlorophenolindophenol (0·15 mM), reduced glutathione (10 mM), and catalase (0·8 mg/ml) in 200 mM TRIS-HCl buffer at pH 7·5. Enzyme activity was determined by collection of $^{14}CO_2$ in Hyamine ® followed by counting in a liquid scintillation spectrometer.

during the purification and also the fact that no activity was observed when the enol form of p-hydroxyphenylpyruvate is used as substrate.

Immunochemical Studies of p-Hydroxyphenylpyruvate Hydroxylase from Human Liver

It has not been established if the tyrosinaemic liver contains a normal amount of an enzyme protein with low or absent catalytic activity or a low concentration of the normal enzyme. In serum pseudocholinesterase deficiency the common variants have normal concentrations of an immunoreactive protein devoid of catalytic activity, whereas one rare variant has no demonstrable immunoreactive protein (Hodgkin *et al.*, 1965). The same has been found with mouse erythrocyte catalase deficiency (Feinstein *et al.*, 1968) and anti-haemophilic globulin deficiency in humans (Feinstein *et al.*, 1969). To examine the situation in hereditary tyrosinaemia, we raised antisera against human p-hydroxyphenylpyruvate hydroxylase in two rabbits. Fig. 9 shows the result of an antigen–antibody

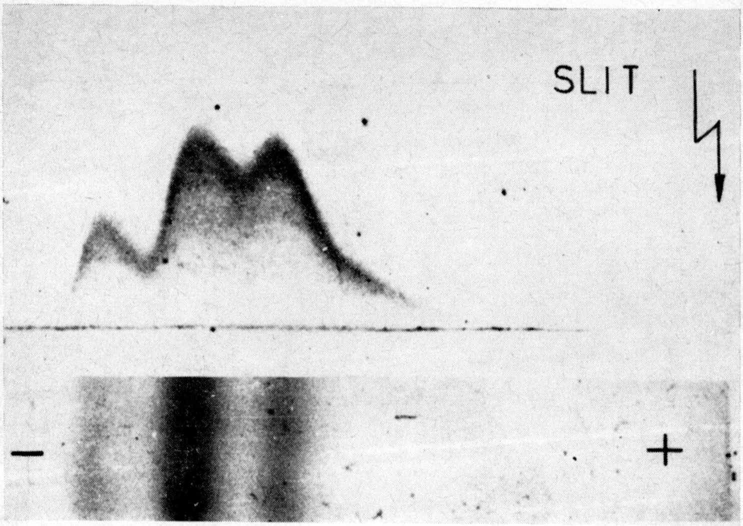

FIG. 9. Antigen–antibody crossed electrophoresis of purified human p-hydroxyphenylpyruvate hydroxylase. The lower part shows the initial electrophoresis in 1 per cent agarose gel in 0·5 M pyridinium chloride buffer at pH 6·3. The upper part shows the subsequent electrophoresis into 1 per cent agarose gel containing rabbit anti-human p-hydroxyphenylpyruvate hydroxylase in 0.075 M diethylbarbiturate buffer at pH 8·6. The gels were stained with coomassie brilliant blue.

crossed electrophoresis (Laurell, 1965) of the material applied to the TEAE-cellulose column shown in Fig. 6. The result of this experiment indicates immunologic identity between the three electrophoretically separable modified forms of the enzyme. On double immunodiffusion according to Ouchterlony (1968) a complete fusion occurred between the precipitation line from the pure enzyme and the precipitation line from a normal liver homogenate. No immunoprecipitate could be observed with a homogenate from the liver of a patient with hereditary tyrosinaemia (Fig. 10). The same result was obtained with the homogenate from another patient. Immunochemical quantitation of the enzyme was performed by the single radial immunodiffusion technique, Fig. 11 (Mancini

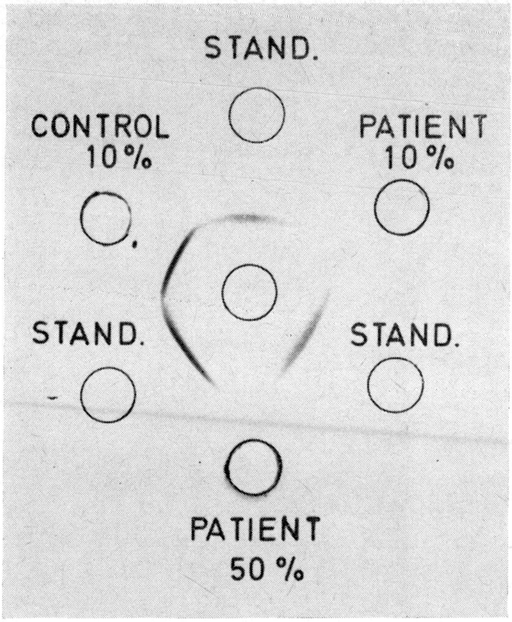

FIG. 10. Immunodiffusion against rabbit anti-human p-hydroxyphenylpyruvate hydroxylase (*center well*) of purified p-hydroxyphenylpyruvate hydroxylase (0·3 μg of enzyme protein, STAND.); 10 per cent homogenate in 0·1 M potassium phosphate buffer, pH 6·5, of normal human liver (0·5 mg of liver tissue, CONTROL 10 per cent); 10 per cent homogenate of liver from a tyrosinaemic patient (PATIENT 10 per cent), and 50 per cent homogenate from the same patient (PATIENT 50 per cent). The gel was stained with coomassie brilliant blue.

et al., 1965). The normal human liver contained about 4 μmoles of the enzyme per kg, calculated on the basis of a molecular weight of 100,000 for the enzyme. No immunoprecipitating material was found (i.e. less than 2 per cent of the control) with homogenates from two patients with hereditary tyrosinaemia. In these patients the residual enzyme activity corresponded to 1 and 2 per cent of the control values. It could be argued that the enzyme exists in a modification which does not form an insoluble antigen–antibody complex. To exclude this possibility a homogenate from a normal liver and the same homogenate *plus* a homogenate from a tyrosinaemic liver was titrated with the antiserum (Fig. 12). There was no difference between the two titration curves. In conclusion, there is at present no indication that significant amounts of a structurally altered enzyme protein with low catalytic activity occurs in hereditary tyrosinaemia.

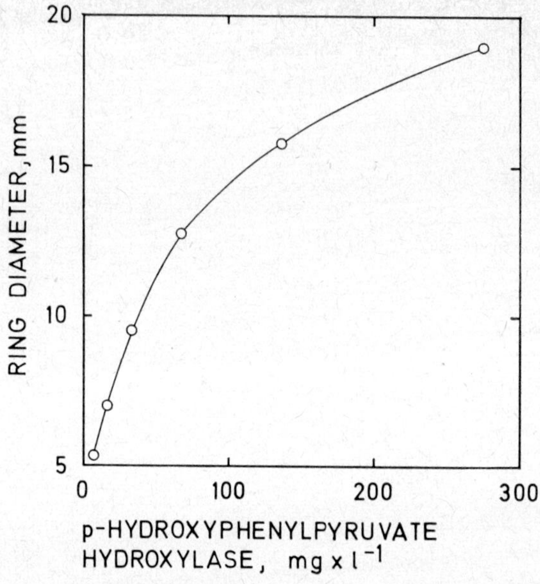

FIG. 11. Determination of p-hydroxyphenylpyruvate hydroxylase by single radial immunodiffusion. The diffusion was carried out for two days at 37°C in 1 per cent agarose gel containing a 1/1000 dilution of serum from a rabbit immunised against human p-hydroxyphenylpyruvate hydroxylase.

Mechanism of Enzymic Formation of Homogentisate from p-Hydroxyphenylpyruvate

The relation between the biochemical abnormalities which have been demonstrated in hereditary tyrosinaemia and the liver cirrhosis which is such a prominent feature of the disease remains obscure. In the metabolism of aromatic compounds intermediates of high tissue toxicity occur, e.g. the epoxides which appear as intermediates in microsomal oxygenation (Jerina *et al.*, 1968, 1970; Selkirk *et al.*, 1971). It cannot be excluded that a reactive intermediate, which is hepatotoxic, is formed in the metabolism of p-hydroxyphenylpyruvate. It is of interest therefore to establish the mechanism for the enzymatic conversion of p-hydroxyphenylpyruvate to homogentisate and also for other possible metabolic pathways for p-hydroxyphenylpyruvate. The formation of homogentisate from p-hydroxyphenylpyruvate involves hydroxylation of the aromatic nucleus combined with oxidative decarboxylation and migration of the side chain (Fig. 13). This reaction shows a certain resemblance to the reactions which occur in a newly discovered class of oxygenases in which 2-ketoglutarate is oxidatively decarboxylated conco-

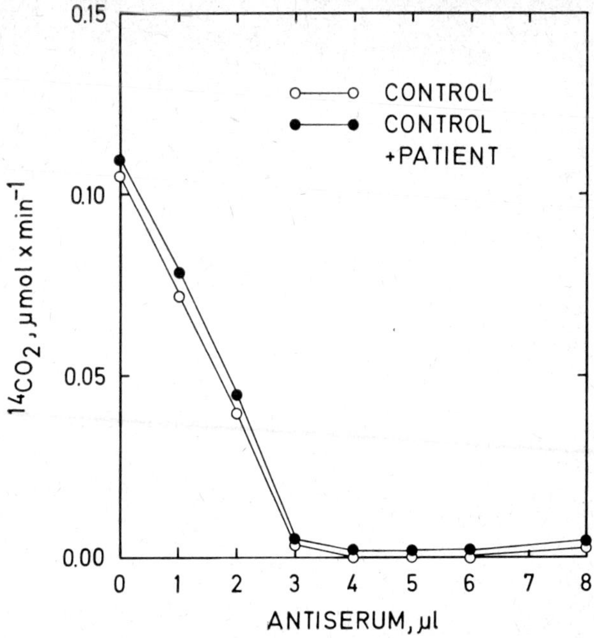

FIG. 12. Titration of human liver homogenate with rabbit anti-human p-hydroxyphenylpyruvate hydroxylase. The experiment was carried out with 250 µl of a normal liver homogenate (5 per cent in 0·1 M potassium phosphate buffer at pH 6·5) and with the same homogenate to which had been added an equal amount of a homogenate of a liver from a case of hereditary tyrosinaemia. After addition of antiserum, the mixture was left at 37°C for 1 hour and then centrifuged. The supernatant was assayed for p-hydroxyphenylpyruvate hydroxylase activity.

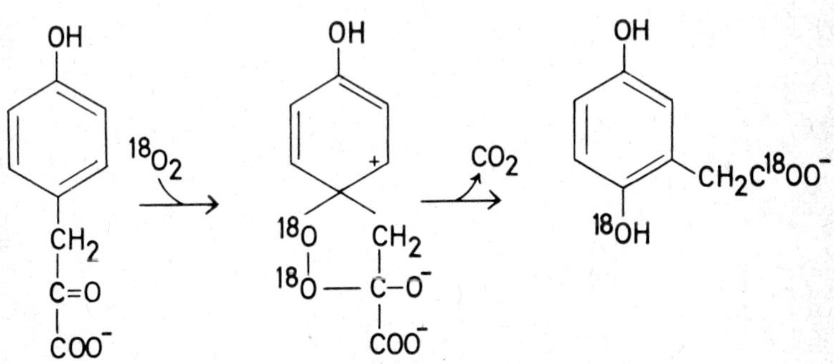

FIG. 13. Proposed intermediate in the formation of homogentisate from p-hydroxyphenylpyruvate.

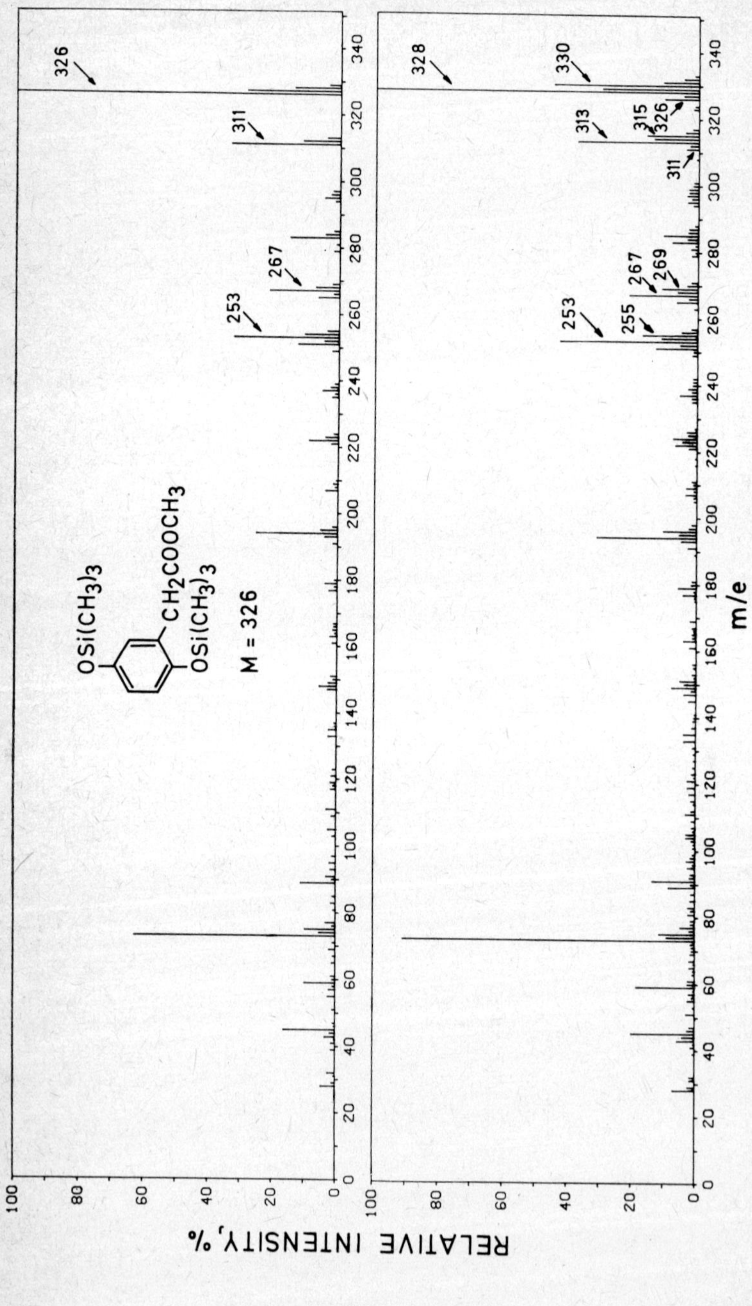

FIG. 14. Mass spectrum of homogentisate formed from p-hydroxyphenylpyruvate in $^{18}O_2$ (*lower*) and of homogentisate from a control incubation (*upper*). The homogentisate was converted to the bistrimethylsilyl ether of the methyl ester and analysed on a LKB 9000 instrument for combined gas chromatography mass-spectrometry.

mitantly with hydroxylation of a substrate. We have previously studied the mechanism of these oxygenases and proposed the formation of an intermediate peroxide (Holme *et al.*, 1968; Lindblad *et al.*, 1969). A similar but cyclic peroxide was therefore envisaged as an intermediate in the formation of homogentisate from p-hydroxyphenylpyruvate (Lindblad *et al.*, 1970). In fact, such an intermediate had already been proposed in 1957 by Goodwin and Witkop (1957). Subsequent experimental data (Yasunobu *et al.*, 1958) were apparently at variance with this mechanism and other alternatives appeared in the literature (Crandall, 1965; Soloway, 1966). With modern mass-spectrometric techniques it has now been possible to show that *both* atoms of an oxygen molecule are incorporated into the formed homogentisate as would be required by the peroxide mechanism (Lindblad *et al.*, 1970) (Figs. 13, 14). We, as well as Goodwin and Witkop, have considered the initial attack of the activated oxygen molecule to be on the carbon atom to be hydroxylated. Alternatively, the initial attack might occur on the keto acid resulting in the formation of a peracid (Fig. 15). It is relevant to this problem that

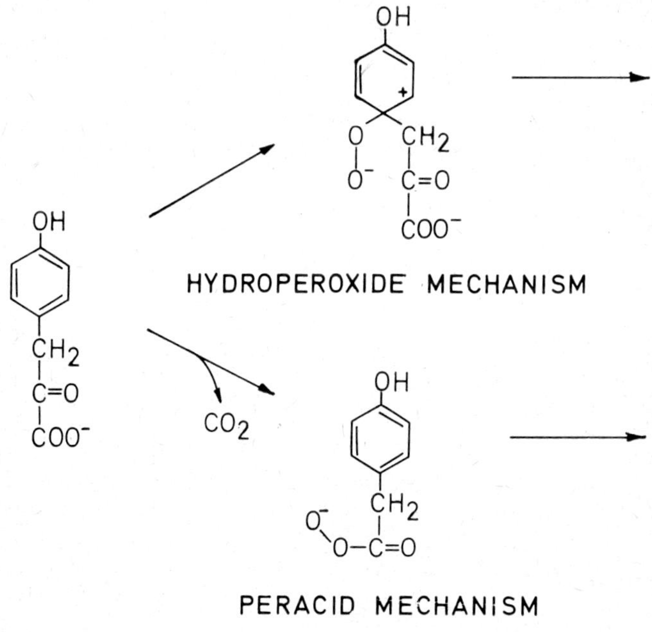

FIG. 15

monopersuccinate cannot replace 2-ketoglutarate for thymine 7-hydroxylase or for γ-butyrobetaine hydroxylase nor is 2-ketoglutarate decarboxylated in the presence of p-hydroxyphenylacetic acid and p-hydroxyphenylpyruvate hydroxylase. 2-Ketoglutarate does not act as a stimulant or inhibitor in the enzyme-catalysed conversion of p-hydroxyphenylpyruvate to homogentisate (unpublished data). Thus, at the present time there is no experimental evidence against the formation of a peroxide intermediate resulting from an initial attack of activated oxygen on the aromatic ring in p-hydroxyphenylpyruvate.

REFERENCES

Bodegård, G., Gentz, J., Lindblad, B., Lindstedt, S. & Zetterström, R. (1969) *Acta paediat. Scand.*, **58**, 37.

Crandall, D. I. (1965) *In* King T. E., Mason, H. S. & Morrison, M. (eds.) *Oxidases and Related Redox Systems*, New York: John Wiley & Sons, Inc., p. 263.

Feinstein, D., Chong, M. N. Y., Casper, C. K. & Rapaport, S. I. (1969) *Science*, **163**, 1071.

Feinstein, R. N., Suter, H. & Jaroslow, B. N. (1968) *Science*, **159**, 638.

Fellman, J. H., Vanbellinghen, P. J., Jones, R. T. & Koler, R. D. (1969) *Biochemistry*, **8**, 615.

Gentz, J., Heinrich, J., Lindblad, B., Lindstedt, S. & Zetterström, R. (1969a) *Acta paediat. Scand.*, **58**, 393.

Gentz, J., Jagenburg, R. & Zetterström, R. (1965) *J. Pediatrics*, **66**, 670.

Gentz, J., Johansson, S., Lindblad, B., Lindstedt, S. & Zetterström, R. (1969b) *Clin. chim. Acta*, **23**, 257.

Gentz, J. & Lindblad, B. (1972) *Scand. J. clin. Lab. Invest.*, *29*, 115.

Gentz, J., Lindblad, B., Lindstedt, S., Levy, L., Shasteen, W. & Zetterström, R. (1967) *Amer. J. Dis. Child.*, **31**, 113.

Gentz, J., Lindblad, B., Lindstedt, S. & Zetterström, R. (1969c) *J. Lab. clin. Med.*, **74**, 185.

Gentz, J., Lindblad, B., Lindstedt, S. & Zetterström, R. (1970) *Pediat. Res.*, **4**, 216.

Gentz, J., Lindblad, B., Lindstedt, S. & Zetterström, R. (1971). In preparation.

Goodwin, S. & Witkop, B. (1957) *J. amer. chem. Soc.*, **79**, 179.

Hager, S. E., Gregerman, R. I. & Know, W. E. (1957) *J. biol. Chem.*, **225**, 935.

Hodgkin, W. E., Giblett, E. R., Levine, H., Bauer, W. & Motulsky, A. G. (1965) *J. clin. Invest.*, **44**, 486.

Holme, E., Lindstedt, G., Lindstedt, S. & Tofft, M. (1968) *Fed. eur. biochem. Soc. Lett.*, **2**, 29.

Jerina, D. M., Daly, J. W., Witkop, B., Zaltzman-Nirenberg, P. & Udenfriend, S. (1968) *J. amer. chem. Soc.*, **90**, 6525.

Jerina, D. M., Daly, J. W., Witkop, B., Zaltzman-Nirenberg, P. & Udenfriend, S. (1970) *Biochemistry*, **9**, 147.

Kang, E. S. & Gerald, P. S. (1970) *J. Pediat.*, **77**, 397.

La Du, B. N. (1967) *Amer. J. Dis. Child.*, **113**, 54.

Laurell, C. B. (1965) *Anal. Biochem.*, **10**, 358.

Lindblad, B. (1971) *Clin. chim. Acta*, *34*, 113.

Lindblad, B., Lindstedt, G. & Lindstedt, S. (1970) *J. amer. chem. Soc.*, **92**, 7446.

Lindblad, B., Lindstedt, S., Olander, B. & Omfeldt, M. (1971) *Acta chem. scand.*, **25**, 329.

Lindblad, B., Lindstedt, G., Tofft, M. & Lindstedt, S. (1969) *J. amer. chem. Soc.*, **91**, 4604.

Mancini, G., Carbonara, A. O. & Heremans, J. F. (1965) *Immunochemistry*, **2**, 235.

Ouchterlony, Ö. (1968) *Handbook of immunodiffusion and immunoelectrophoresis*, Michigan: Ann Arbor Science Publishers, Inc.

Selkirk, J. K., Huberman, E. & Heidelberger, C. (1971) *Biochem. biophys. Res. Commun.*, **43**, 1010.
Soloway, A. H. (1966) *J. theor. Biol.*, **13**, 100.
Taniguchi, K., Kappe, T. & Armstrong, M. D. (1964) *J. biol. Chem.*, **239**, 3389.
Waalkes, T. P. & Udenfriend, S. (1957) *J. Lab. clin. Med.*, **50**, 733.
Yasunobu, K., Tanaka, T., Know, W. E. & Mason, H. S. (1958) *Fed. Proc.*, **17**, 340.
Yphantis, D. A. (1964) *Biochemistry*, **3**, 297.
Zannoni, V. G. & La Du, B. N. (1956) *Fed. Proc.*, **15**, 391.
Zannoni, V. G. & La Du, B. N. (1959) *J. biol. Chem.*, **234**, 2925.

DISCUSSION
(on the Papers by Professor La Du and Professor Lindstedt)

Seakins (*London*). Recently at the Hospital for Sick Children we were faced with the following problem: should we place an infant with many features of classical tyrosinosis on a diet low in phenylalanine and tyrosine. Before a decision was reached the child responded well to a low-protein diet. This patient showed an odd phenylalanine/tyrosine response following a load of 100 mg/kg of phenylalanine which indicated a delayed-conversion of phenylalanine to tyrosine and of tyrosine to p-hydroxyphenylpyruvic acid. Professor Lindstedt, do you find phenylalanine load tests of value in distinguishing the transient form of hypertyrosenaemia from tyrosinosis? Dr La Du, are low prothrombin times an indication of tyrosinosis?

La Du (*New York*). One of the primary differences between the serious disease hereditary tyrosinaemia and the transitory form is the bleeding problem. Bleeding does not seem to occur in the transitory form of hypertyrosinaemia. If the child has a bleeding problem then most likely it is to be of the hereditary type, bleeding does not occur in transitory hypertyrosinaemia even though this goes on for several weeks.

Lindstedt (*Gothenburg*). I think you will find the same type of response to a loading test in these two conditions. We have measured the excretion of δ-ALA* in only one case of transient tyrosinaemia; the excretion fell within the normal range. In all cases of hereditary tyrosinaemia we have found an increased excretion of δ-ALA, often higher than in acute intermittent porphyria. This has to be looked into more systematically in cases of transitory tyrosinaemia.

Black (*Sheffield*). Professor La Du, what in your view is the significance of the occurrence of hepatoma in hereditary tyrosinaemia? Do you think some of the phenolic compounds are carcinogenic?

La Du. I cannot give an explanation because we do not know whether these aromatic compounds bind to tissue proteins in the way we are suggesting. Perhaps you are thinking about the possibility of direct

*δ-ALA = δ-amino laevulic acid.

interaction of epoxide type intermediates; when protecting sulphydryl groups are reduced these could react with either nucleic acid or the sulphydryl groups of amino acids. It is possible that one might get some of the same changes that occur with other covalently linked derivatives of the type. This is one of the reasons why we suspect it may be another kind of liver enzyme deficiency which makes the liver more vulnerable to these metabolites which ordinarily could be handled.

Brenton (*London*). Professor Lindstedt, in view of the report by Rimington (*Clinical Science*, **16**, 517, 1957) on a patient with hepatoma and porphyria do you think that the increase δ-aminolaevulinic acid excretion in your patients with tyrosinosis is peculiar to them or may it occur in hepatomas or liver disease of other aetiologies. The incidence of cutaneous porphyria is also relevant here.

Lindstedt. I remember that case—a lady 80 years old who recovered completely on removal of a hepatoma. I do not know whether the incidence of liver cancer is higher in this group compared with liver cirrhosis in general. In alcoholic cirrhosis liver cancer appears to be quite common. These patients do not excrete increased amounts of δ-ALA—as seems to be characteristic for hereditary tyrosinaemia.

Berry (*Cincinnati*). Have you measured p-hydroxyphenylpyruvic acid oxidase in untreated galactosaemia? In this disease biochemical abnormalities of tyrosine metabolism are similar to those found in hereditary tyrosinaemia. Can you speculate about the mechanism of the abnormal tyrosine metabolism in galactosaemia?

La Du. Not specifically—it seems that PHPP oxidase is an enzyme which is unusually easily inhibited. It can be inhibited both by—SH binding compounds and by peroxides. It is susceptible to so many types of inhibition. Once inhibited the accumulation of substrate perpetuates the defect so I think it is just an indicator enzyme.

I wonder whether Professor Lindstedt considers there to be stronger support for this inhibition theory of PHPP oxidase than to the enzyme being deficient in hereditary tyrosinaemia.

Lindstedt. Immunological studies have shown that there is no enzyme protein present in these patients, or at least very little. With the inhibition theory you have to postulate that the inhibitor-enzyme complex is eliminated very rapidly, somehow like haptoglobin. There is no evidence for that.

One may speculate as you did Dr La Du, that the increased concentration of PHPP may act as substrate for other enzymes, for example, microsomal hydroxylases, and in that way may give rise to liver toxins.

Eldjarn (*Oslo*). The brilliant presentations by La Du and Lindstedt poses the question of how to promote systematic co-operation in the study of these relatively rare disorders—perhaps a task for this society. Clearly, the enzyme activity studies presented here can scarcely be compared: in some the disappearance of the substrate is measured, in others the formation of products, some are referred to mg of tissue, others to nitrogen content, dry weight, DNA, various reference enzymes. I believe progress would be facilitated if we did not aim at what may be compared to individual collections of rare stamps! Would it be possible for this Society to establish reference centres—or persons—for the various rare inborn errors?

Raine (*Birmingham*). I would like to draw together a number of intellectual difficulties we have experienced, some of which have been referred to in this discussion.

We have had otherwise healthy patients who persistently excreted tyrosine metabolites and who were detected as a result of the neonatal screening programme. We have had one patient who died in infancy and who had the pathological features of 'tyrosinosis'. We are presented with neonates with frank liver disease, so-called neonatal hepatitis, and also older children with frank liver disease, both of whom may show an abnormality of tyrosine, with or without an abnormality of methionine in either blood or urine, or both. We also have two patients with a primary methionine abnormality similar to that first described by Perry *et al.* (*Pediatrics*, **36**, 236, 1965) and which I believe these authors have been prematurely persuaded were really cases of 'tyrosinosis'. Other cases present with hepatomegaly, with or without jaundice, such as the galactosaemic infants excreting tyrosine metabolites referred to by Dr Berry.

Generally it is not possible to make a confident diagnosis in any of these categories without following the patient to termination or remission, and it would seem to be very valuable if this whole clinical range could be deliberately studied by those able to perform these discriminating enzyme studies, as, without this, it will remain extremely difficult to discover which biochemical features are primary and which secondary.

Bickel (*Heidelberg*). Professor La Du, one of our patients with hereditary tyrosinaemia showed considerable improvement on a tyrosine-restricted diet. His rickets and renal function improved markedly. Have you any up-to-date information about the efficacy of this diet? A marked and reproducible beneficial effect would suggest, though not prove, that tyrosine is the prime noxious agent in this disease.

La Du. That is a very difficult question to answer. From what I can understand from the literature and talking to a number of people about this it does seem that biochemically and clinically the renal reabsorption defects are considerably improved by putting children on a low tyrosine and phenylalanine diet; also there may be a delay in the progression of cirrhosis changes in such patients. It seems to be the accepted experimental approach to therapy to-day and I would not want to discourage anyone from using that treatment.

I am not convinced that the basic defect is really corrected in this way. But from assays of the PHPP oxidase it does look as if the level increases with such treatment which means we still have to think about the deficiency of PHPP oxidase being perpetuated by some inhibitory mechanism which may be removed or reduced by the low diet. The children treated in this way may look better biochemically, they seem to be very precariously balanced, minor infections will throw them out of line. They seem to die from infectious diseases having very little resistance to them; therefore, I am still not convinced that we have explored the aetiology and pathology in this disease to the point when we can say that we have done any more than treat the biochemical symptoms of the disease and have observed some obvious clinical improvement.

I wonder whether a diet which would provide more sulphydryl groups would be of some benefit for example. It seems that this disease should be explored in a more general way and it may be you are perfectly right in that this being the major defect, I do not know how to relate this to the methionine problem.

There are interrelationships between mathionine and tyrosine metabolism which need to be worked out and Dr Perry has started a line there. It would be nice to tell clinicians from an enzymology stand point what is wrong and what should be done.

I am sure that both of us would be very happy to assay any biopsy sample that comes in, we do this regularly. It so happens that no patients with galactosaemia have been examined and liver samples sent to us. I do not think that we have ever turned down a liver sample.

Lombeck (*Dusseldorf*). A female patient of ours, aged 12 months, with hereditary tyrosinaemia died 4 days after being given a phenylalanine load of 200 mg/kg. She had been treated with phenylalanine and tyrosine restricted diet.

Lindstedt. I do not think it was the loading test which caused death. As I mentioned some patients have had bad episodes with hypertension, pains and paralysis of respiratory muscles. It is not clear what initiates these crises, but it does not appear to be, for instance, an excessive protein intake.

Curtius (*Zurich*). I have a question for Dr Lindblad, was the concentration of adrenaline and nor-adrenaline also elevated during the loading test with phenylalanine or was it perhaps decreased.

Lindblad (*Gothenburg*). I do not think that we ever measured it.

Watts (*Harrow*). It seems to me that Dr La Du may be emphasising the possibility that the basic lesion is perhaps due to inhibition of p-hydroxyphenylpyruvic acid oxidase by a toxic metabolite. However, Dr Lindstedt has shown immunochemical evidence that the protein is lacking. If this is so the inhibition would have to be one of protein synthesis affecting one enzyme protein selectively. This seems unlikely to me and would in no way conform to the way in which protein synthesis in general is inhibited, for example, in experimental studies with cyclohexamide and puromycin. The evidence presented by Dr Lindstedt, appears to favour the concept that lack of p-hydroxyphenylpyruvic acid oxidase is the primary enzyme defect. Would the speakers care to comment?

La Du. There are several ways of looking at this, you might think that when the enzyme is inhibited its rate of degradation is faster and so the steady state concentration of the enzyme would be reduced when it undergoes this inhibition.

I am not sure in your immunochemical assays whether you tested substrate inhibited enzyme to see whether this reacted as the native enzyme does. The problem of the forms of the enzyme is interesting, we have some data suggesting that there is more than one form of the enzyme. It is a very peculiar enzyme in that sodium dodecyl sulphate can split the enzyme into fragments with smaller molecular weight, we have done this with the same techniques as you have and in the split form it loses its ability to catalyse the oxidation of phenylpyruvic acid. It does seem that this is reversible, whereas the PHPP oxidase is still preserved in the smaller molecular weight form. It also appears that copper is a cofactor in PHPP oxidase activity and iron is involved in the oxidation of phenylpyruvic acid. It is therefore a peculiar enzyme.

Until we learn more about the form of the enzyme, its stability and degradation I think it will be hard to decide which theory is the most important. It could be that its turnover is changed when it is inhibited as well as when it is present in reduced amounts.

Lindstedt. I agree that there are interesting properties of the enzyme, it has to be purified and studied in more detail. So far we can say that there is no immunological evidence for the presence of enzymatic protein whether this is because of a complex with an inhibitor being rapidly eliminated or not, I do not know. I have no opinion on this.

Eldjarn. I am, of course, exceedingly happy to hear that the two speakers are willing to assay enzyme activities in samples sent to them. May I ask in this connection if they have assayed samples from each other. If they have done so, and if their data agree, then I shall feel much safer in accepting that we are talking about the same thing and that similar disorders occur on both sides of the Atlantic.

A VARIANT OF BRANCHED-CHAIN KETOACIDURIA

by

SELMA E. SNYDERMAN*

CONTINUED investigation of branched-chain ketoaciduria (maple syrup urine disease) suggests that this disorder follows the same pattern that has become apparent in a number of other metabolic disorders. First, there is the recognition and elucidation of the most dramatic form of the disease, which in time is referred to as the classic type, and then variations are encountered which are not as severe either in their clinical manifestations or in the degree of biochemical abnormality.

The salient features of classic maple syrup urine disease are those of a rapidly fatal disease including feeding disorders, loss of reflexes, alternating periods of hypo and hypertonia, convulsions, respiratory arrest, coma and death. This downhill course can be extremely rapid, with death occurring as early as the second week of life (Snyderman *et al.*, 1964). At the other extreme, is the intermittent type in which clinical symptoms only appear as the result of some stress such as an intercurrent illness. The site of the metabolic block is the same in both forms of the disease, a failure of oxidative decarboxylation of the keto acid derivatives of the branched-chain amino acids (Fig. 1); the severity of the clinical manifestations is apparently related to the degree of enzyme activity. There is no detectable activity in the classical form while there is a significant amount of activity in the intermittent form. The variant to be described seems to be between those two extremes of the disease process.

Thomas A. was referred to us at 18 months of age with a history that went back to early infancy. He had been hospitalised on at least three occasions because of extreme irritability, poor feeding, and vomiting. He was examined by a paediatric neurologist at 13 months of age because of episodes of unconsciousness, seizures, and ataxia which first became apparent when he started to walk. This examination revealed evidences of motor retardation, muscle weakness, and ataxia. All of the diagnostic tests performed at this time including a pneumoencephalogram, a brain scan, and an electroencephalogram were within normal limits. During a subsequent examination at 16 months of age because of increasing ataxia, lethargy, and a period of unconsciousness that lasted 24 hours, the urine first had the unmistakable odour of maple syrup, and the child was referred for further study.

* Supported by Project No. 317, Maternal and Child Health Service, Department of Health, Education and Welfare.

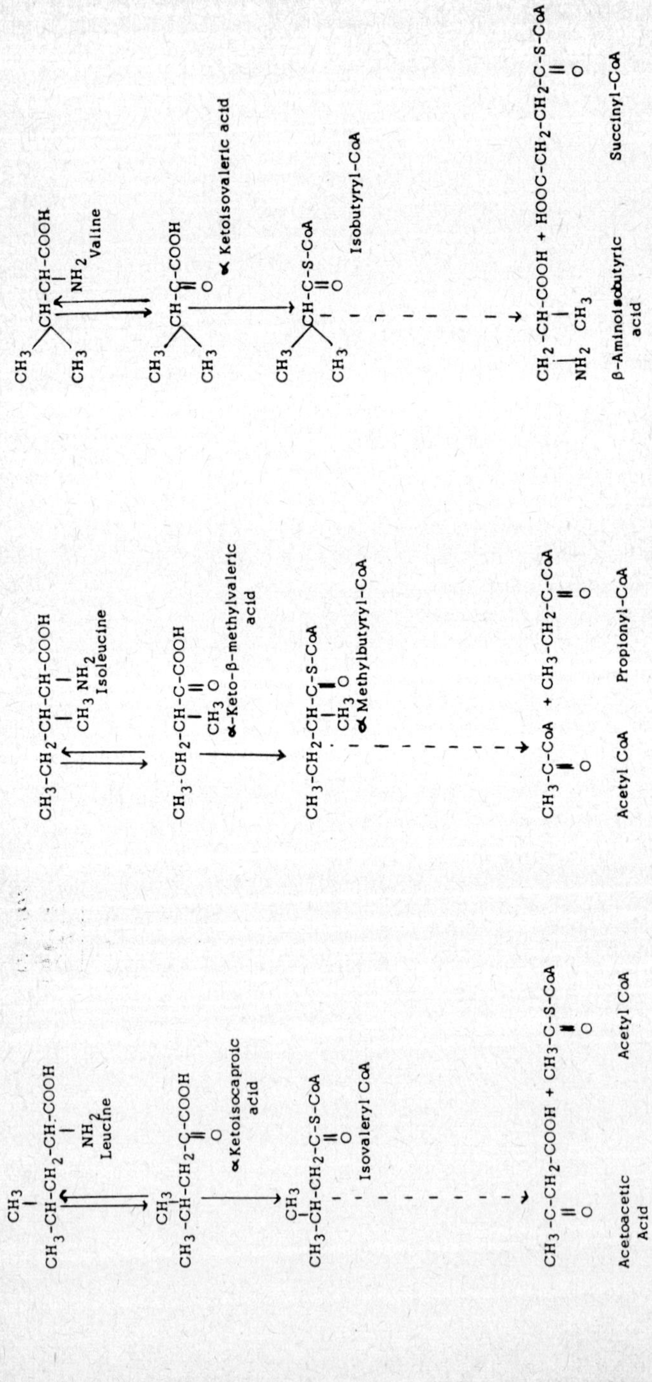

FIG. 1. The metabolic pathways of the branched-chain amino acids.

Because of difficulties in the immediate transfer of this boy to our hospital, we recommended the institution of a low-protein diet in the interim. This resulted in alleviation of the ataxia and a cessation of the seizures. At the time of his admission to Bellevue Hospital 1 month later, there were no abnormal neurologic findings except for the obvious retardation; at the age of 19 months, he functioned at the 9-month level. The plasma branched-chain amino acids were normal, there was no abnormal excretion of the keto acid derivatives of the branched-chain amino acids, and there was no maple syrup odour. All other clinical and biochemical investigations were within normal limits.

A trial of a more usual protein intake for this age (2 g/kg) resulted in a prompt biochemical relapse. Branched-chain ketoaciduria appeared within four days followed by elevation of the plasma branched-chain amino acids (Fig. 2). The child became irritable and quite ataxic. He was

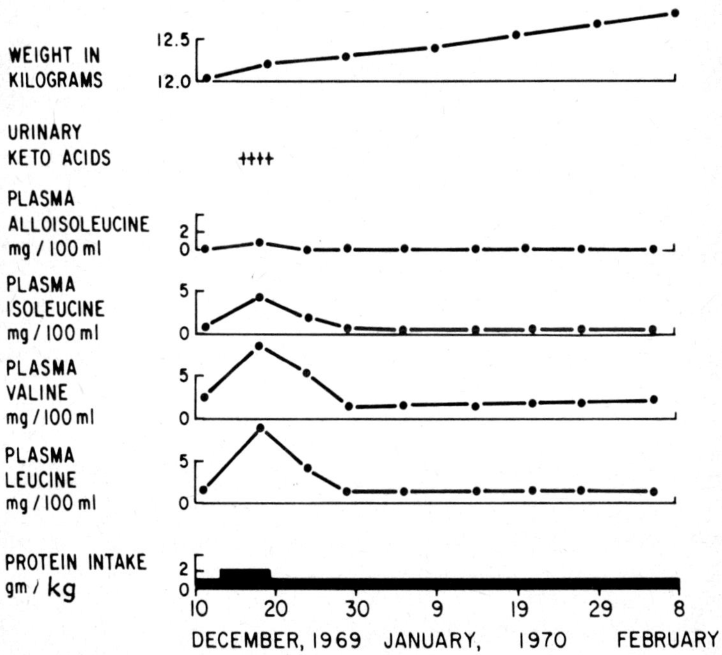

FIG. 2. Protocol of patient TA, illustrating the biochemical relapse that occurred when the protein intake was increased to 2 g/kg/day.

then put back on the low-protein intake of 1 g/kg with prompt clinical and biochemical remission. This diet provided three to four times the quantities of branched-chain amino acids tolerated by classical maple syrup urine disease patients of the same age. The clinical course and the ease with which biochemical control could be achieved with higher branched-chain amino acid intake suggested that this was a variant form of the disease and that some decarboxylase activity was present. This impression was confirmed by enzyme assays performed in the laboratory of Dr Joseph Dancis on cultures of skin fibroblasts; activity of each of the branched-chain decarboxylases was in the range of 5 per cent of normal.

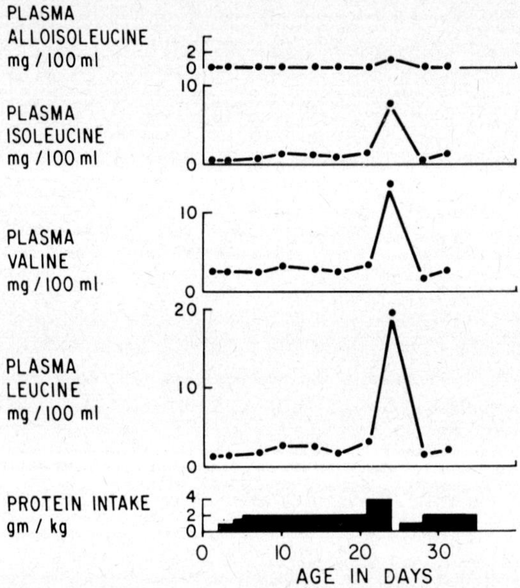

FIG. 3. Protocol of patient MA illustrating the influence of an increase of protein intake on the plasma branched-chain amino acid levels.

A newborn brother of this boy also apparently has the same variant of the disease. He first came under our care at 10 hours of age at which time the plasma amino acids were normal and there was no excessive ketoaciduria. Protein intake was gradually increased to 2g/kg during the first days of life without the appearance of either chemical or clinical abnormalities. A trial of increased protein intake to 4 g/kg at 21 days of age resulted in the prompt appearance of biochemical abnormalities and clinical symptoms (Fig. 3). The baby fed poorly, vomited, cried continuously and was very irritable. All protein was removed from the diet for 24 hours, it was then reintroduced in a stepwise fashion until it was ascertained that he again tolerated 2 g/kg. He has been maintained on this protein intake since then, has not manifested any biochemical relapse, and now at 8 months of age, is neurologically intact, has not had any seizures and has a normal developmental pattern. Study of the enzyme activity of his skin fibroblasts revealed activity in the same range as that of his brother.

The presence of some degree of enzyme activity in these children, suggested that some benefit might be derived from massive doses of thiamine since this vitamin does participate in the first step of branched-chain keto acid decarboxylation (Fig. 4).

α-Keto acid + (thiamine-PP) $\rightarrow$ (active aldehyde-thiamine-PP) + CO_2
(Active aldehyde-thiamine-PP) + (lip-S_2) $\rightarrow$ (acyl-S-lip-S) + (thiamine-PP)
(Acyl-S-lip-SH) + CoA-SH $\rightarrow$ acyl-S-CoA + (lip$(SH)_2$)

FIG. 4

FIG. 4. The steps in the decarboxylation of the keto acid derivatives of the branched-chain amino acids illustrating the role of thiamine and lipoic acid.

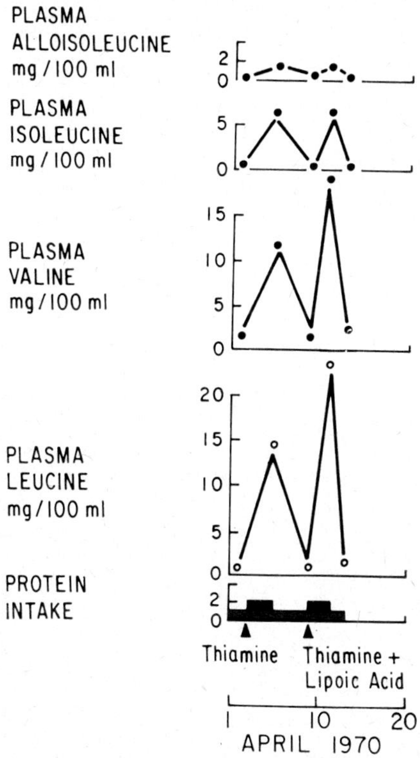

FIG. 5. The effect of a large dose of thiamine and of thiamine plus lipoic acid on the course of patient TA.

This therapeutic trial was made in the older child. He was given the protein intake previously associated with biochemical relapse and large doses of thiamine, 100 mg parenterally daily. Biochemical relapse occurred promptly accompanied by the appearance of ataxia. After return of the plasma amino acids to normal by the usual dietary restriction, a second therapeutic trial of thiamine and lipoic acid was also unsuccessful (Fig. 5). Since this attempt, Scriver (1971) has published a short account of successful thiamine therapy on one case. This may represent still another variant of the disease.

In an attempt to ascertain the tolerance of this child for the branched-chain amino acids, loads of each were given (Figs. 6, 7, 8). The expected response was seen—a greater plasma elevation of the amino acid which persisted for a longer period of time than the same load in a normal individual. In addition, a load of any one of the three amino acids resulted in a plasma elevation of the other two branched-chain amino acids as well. This effect was most striking and persistent in the case of leucine loading. Quantitative determination of the keto acid urinary excretion before and after the loading suggested that this was the result of some interference with decarboxylation. There was virtually no keto acid excretion during the control period, but appreciable quantities after each load. More α-ketoisocaproic acid was excreted after the leucine load and

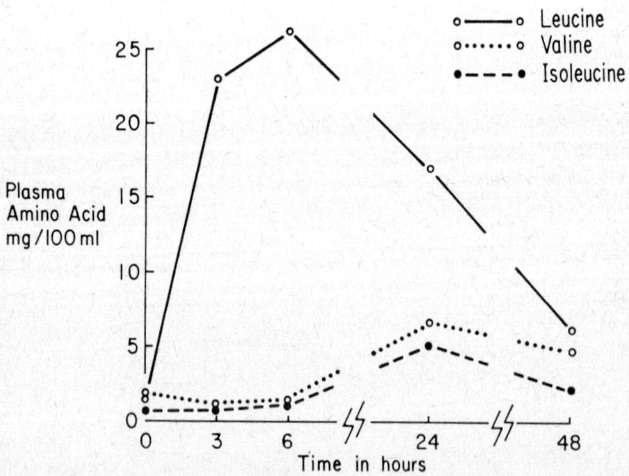

FIG. 6. The effect of a load of leucine on the plasma branched-chain amino acids (patient TA).

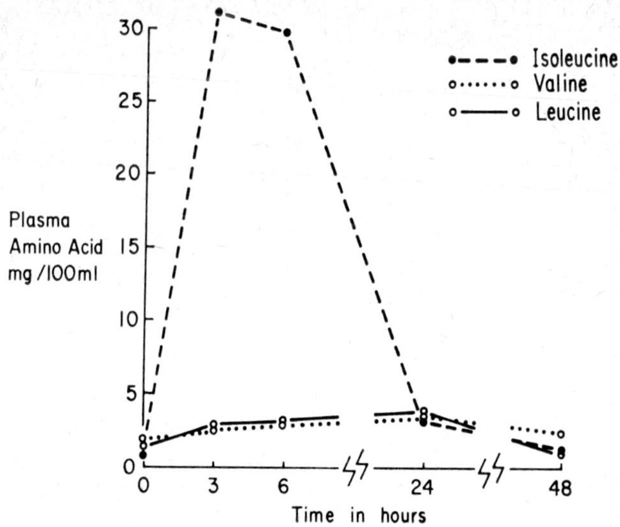

FIG. 7. The effect of a load of isoleucine on the plasma branched-chain amino acids (patient TA).

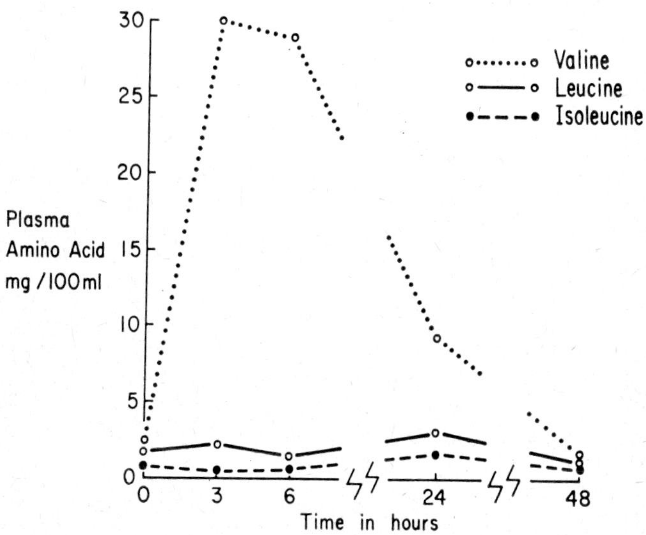

FIG. 8. The effect of a load of valine on the plasma branched-chain amino acids (patient TA).

it was accompanied by greater excretion of the derivatives of the other branched-chain amino acids (Fig. 9).

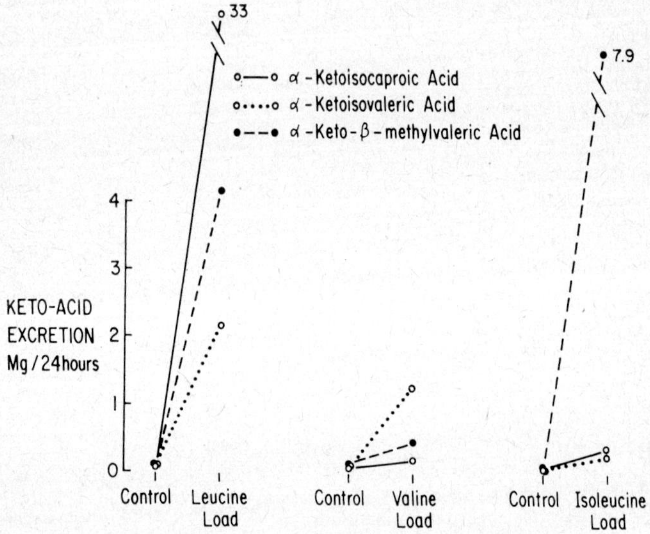

FIG. 9. The increase in keto acid urinary excretion as a result of a load of each of the branched-chain amino acids (patient TA).

This effect of leucine loading on the plasma levels of the other two branched-chain amino acids is different from the results obtained with the normal control subject. In the normal, a load of one of the branched-chain amino acids is followed by a fall in the levels of the other two branched-chain amino acids (Fig. 10). Again, the results after leucine loading are the most striking. Increased excretion of keto acid derivatives does not occur in the normal as a result of loading with the branched-chain amino acids. The mechanism of these plasma alterations in the normal has interested us for some time. They are not the result of interference with gastrointestinal absorption since they are manifest as soon as one hour after loading and while the subject is in the fasting state. They are not the result of alterations in renal tubular reabsorption; the urinary excretion of valine and isoleucine is depressed after a load of leucine and an elevated excretion would be necessary to explain the fall in their plasma levels (Snyderman *et al.*, 1968). The remaining hypothesis, that the depressed plasma levels of isoleucine and valine are the result of metabolic stimulation by excess leucine was confirmed by a study with rats (Phansalkar *et al.*, 1970). Rats were given a dose of uniformly labelled ^{14}C isoleucine, and the expired $^{14}CO_2$ was measured. After this rate of excretion had become constant, a load of leucine was adminis-

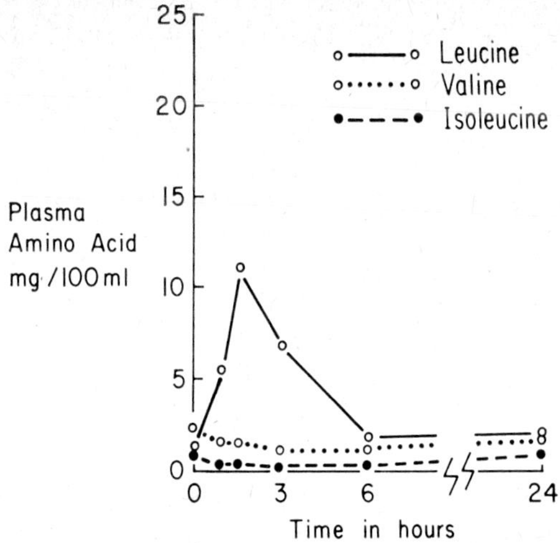

FIG. 10. The effect of a load of leucine on the plasma branched-chain amino acids in the normal individual.

tered. There was a marked increase in the amount of $^{14}CO_2$ expired by every rat that received the leucine load. The results obtained were statistically significant (Fig. 11).

This enhanced metabolism of isoleucine and valine after leucine loading in the normal, emphasises the abnormality in the variant of branched-chain ketoaciduria. The exact significance of this abnormality is not presently apparent. It has been suggested that there is inactivity of only one enzyme in branched-chain ketoaciduria, that the keto acid accumulation of one amino acid interferes with decarboxylation of the other two. The results in this case are certainly consistent with this theory. However, the study of enzyme activity of this child's fibroblasts, and that in classical maple syrup urine disease, revealed involvement of all three decarboxylases. These observations indicate that the biochemical derangement may be due to a combination of both of these factors.

SUMMARY

An unusual variant of maple syrup urine disease is described. The clinical manifestations included retardation, ataxia, convulsions and one episode of coma. Elevation of plasma branched-chain amino acids and ketoaciduria were present on a normal diet and disappeared promptly when the protein intake was restricted. Markedly depressed enzyme activity of all three decarboxylases could be demonstrated. In contrast to

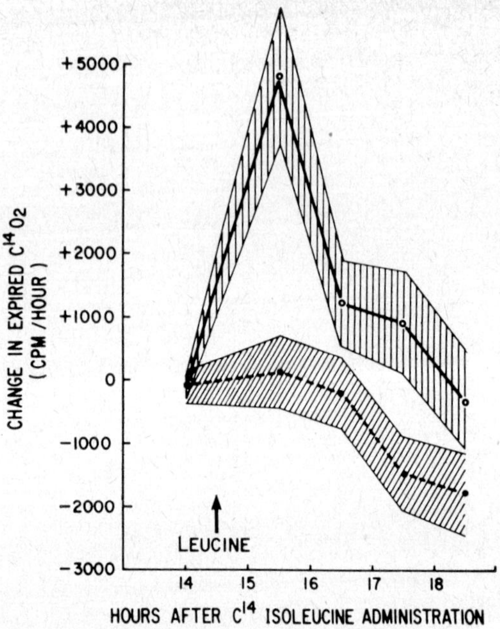

FIG. 11. The increase in $^{14}CO_2$ production resulting from a load of L-leucine to rats previously given L-isoleucine (U)-^{14}C: (...) average control and (—) average experimental result; (shaded areas), one standard error above and below the average.

the normal, loading with one of the branched-chain amino acids resulted in the plasma elevation of all three and in the excretion of their keto acid derivatives.

REFERENCES

PHANSALKAR, S. V., NORTON, P. M., HOLT, L. E., JR. & SNYDERMAN, S. E. (1970) *Proc. Soc. exp. Biol. Med.*, **134**, 262.

SCRIVER, C. R., CLOW, C. L., MACKENZIE, S. & DELVIN, E. (1971) *Lancet*, **1**, 310.

SNYDERMAN, S. E., NORTON, P. M., ROITMAN, E. & HOLT, L. E. JR. (1964) *Pediatrics* **34**, 454.

SNYDERMAN, S. E., HOLT, L. E. JR, NORTON, P. M. & ROITMAN, E. (1968) in Leathem, J. H. (ed.) *Protein Nutrition and Free Amino Acid Patterns*, New Brunswick, N. J.: Rutgers University Press, p. 19.

DISCUSSION
(of the Paper by Dr Snyderman)

Bickel (*Heidelberg*). I cannot see the distinction between the variant form of MSUD which you have just described and the 'intermittent' form, which we have observed in one patient over the past six years. This boy fits exactly into the pattern of the intermittent form as described in the literature. He was mildly mentally retarded before being given a protein-restricted diet. He is now normal but is very sensitive in his clinical and biochemical manifestations to an increase in his daily protein intake.

Snyderman (*New York*). In the intermittent form, biochemical abnormalities and symptoms occur only when there is some stress such as febrile illness. Dietary therapy is not necessary except during these periods. The child I am describing had increased levels of his branched-chain amino acids and the appearance of clinical symptoms whenever he exceeded the prescribed protein intake. There is also a difference in the amount of enzyme present.

Bickel. How constant was the increase in the blood level of the other branched-chain amino acids if the level of one of them was raised by loading? I seem to remember that in our last patient with MSUD the blood level of isoleucine and valine often *dropped* when the leucine concentration in the blood increased.

Snyderman. We have observed a fall in the plasma levels of the other branched-chain amino acids when a load of the third was given in the normal individual. However, when a sufficient load is given to the child with MSUD, there is usually an elevation of the other two branched-chain amino acids.

Gerritsen (*Madison*). A paper on 'Biochemical Studies on a Variant of MSUD in a 19-year-old Female' was recently published (Fischer, M. H. & Gerritsen, T., *Pediatrics*, **48**, 795, 1971). Their patient had a full scale IQ of 76, was physically in good health, but excreted large amounts of branched-chain α-keto acids in the urine. Interestingly, more than 75 per cent of these consisted of α-keto-β-methylvaleric acid, while in classic MSUD more than 50 per cent of the excreted α-keto acids consists of α-ketoisocaproic acid. On a normal diet, the patient's plasma levels of leucine, isoleucine and valine were only about 2 to 4 times normal, as compared with up to 40 times normal levels in classic MSUD. On a high protein intake these levels increased to no more than 4 to 8 times normal and the excretion of branched-chain amino acids and branched-chain α-keto acid could be increased. Branched-chain α-keto acid dehydrogenase activities in the peripheral leucocytes and in skin fibroblast were almost zero and comparable to the levels found in a case of classic MSUD.

It looks to me that the variant discussed by Dr Snyderman is different from our case, and also different from the variant reported by Schulman *et al.*, 1970 (*Amer. J. Med.* **49**, 118).

Cusworth (*London*). Dr Snyderman, is administration of non-metabolisable amino acids to these infants hazardous?

Snyderman. The loads of amino acids were not large enough to be considered hazardous to these children who did have some enzyme activity present. They were also very carefully monitored throughout theprocedure.

Cusworth. With reference to the interrelationship of the enzymes metabolising the branched-chain amino acids, what is the significance of the observations by Snyderman *et al.* (1968)* that in normal subjects restriction of intake of one branched-chain amino acid leads to a marked increase in the other two. Is this relevant to the difficulties in establishing dietary control in some 'classical' MSUD patients—it seems that isoleucine levels will remain high if leucine intake is too low.

Snyderman. This interrelationship between the branched-chain amino acids is dependent on the presence of the enzymes necessary for their metabolism. I do not think it is pertinent in MSUD where there is complete absence of decarboxylase activity.

Cusworth. With regard to Dr Gerritsen's patient—although enzyme activity may be 'immeasurable', there may in fact be a small amount there, sufficient to deal with a normal load. This may be a general, almost philosophical, point not restricted to MSUD. For example, in homocystinuria, enzyme activity may be too low to measure. Treatment with pyridoxine leads to biochemical improvement, but enzyme activity remains 'immeasurable'. There may, however, have been a small, 'immeasurable' rise in enzyme activity which enables the patient to cope with his normal dietary load.

* 'Effect of high and low intakes of Individual Amino Acid on the Plasma Aminogram *in Protein Nutrition and Free Amino Acid Patterns*, ed. J. H. Leathem, Rutgers University Press, New Brunswick, N.J., p. 19.

BENZOIC ACIDURIA IN CHRONIC PSYCHOSES

by

THOMAS L. PERRY, SHIRLEY HANSEN AND DONNA LESK

Introduction

IN man benzoic acid is normally detoxified in the liver by conjugation with glycine to form hippuric acid. Considerable quantities of benzoic acid are ingested in a normal diet. The compound occurs naturally in many fruits and berries, particularly in cranberries, prunes and plums. Sodium benzoate is added as a preservative (in concentrations ranging from 0·05 to 0·10 per cent) to a wide variety of commercially prepared foods. Among these are carbonated and still beverages, fruit juices and fruit cocktails, pickles and relishes, jams and jellies, catsup, pie and pastry fillings, marinated fish, and salted margarine (Furia, 1968). Although dietary sources account for most of the benzoic acid that is metabolised to hippuric acid in man, small amounts of benzoic acid also are produced endogenously from phenylalanine. On a synthetic diet free of benzaldehyde and benzoic acid, normal adults still excrete 60 to 150 mg of hippuric acid daily (Armstrong, 1963).

The synthesis of hippuric acid in mammals requires the action of two enzyme systems, both of which are found only within mitochondria in liver and kidney. Benzoic acid is first converted to benzoyl adenylate by pyrophosphate exchange with adenosine triphosphate, and the adenylate moiety is then exchanged for co-enzyme A to produce benzoyl CoA. These two reactions are catalysed by a thiokinase. Finally, benzoyl CoA reacts with glycine to yield hippuric acid and free co-enzyme A. This last reaction is catalysed by the enzyme glycine N-acylase (E.C. 2.3.1.13) (Schachter & Taggart, 1954a). Free benzoate has not been reported as a normal constituent of human urine, and it generally has been assumed that benzoic acid is completely metabolised to hippuric acid in healthy individuals.

We recently discovered three patients with chronic schizophrenia in a mental hospital in Canada who excreted large amounts of benzoic acid in their urine (Perry, Hansen, Diamond, Melançon & Lesk, 1971). This led us to screen a population of chronically hospitalised psychiatric patients in Norway, and a second population of control subjects free of mental or neurological disease in Canada, for this biochemical abnormality. Our studies suggest that a small minority of psychotic adults may have an intermittent impairment of their ability to conjugate benzoic acid with glycine, and that this biochemical defect may possibly be causally related to the mental dysfunction in these patients.

Subjects and Methods

Subjects

Morning urine specimens were collected after an overnight fast from 307 psychiatric patients (208 men and 99 women) who were hospitalised at the Dikemark Sykehus. This hospital cares for chronically mentally ill adults from the city of Oslo, Norway. All patients living on certain wards were studied, without attempting to include or exclude any diagnostic categories. Although a majority of the patients were believed to have some form of schizophrenia, the study also included patients with depressive and senile psychoses, as well as patients whose mental disease followed a head injury or cerebrovascular accident. Twenty-nine per cent of the patients were aged over 60 years.

Since arrangements could not be made to study a Norwegian control population, morning urines were collected from a control group of 510 mentally normal subjects living in Vancouver, Canada. These included 239 men and 271 women, 31 per cent of whom were aged over 60 years. As far as could be determined, the diets consumed by the Norwegian psychiatric in-patients and the Canadian control subjects were both nutritionally adequate, and they contained comparable amounts of benzoate.

Screening for hippuric acid

Urine specimens were frozen promptly after collection and were stored at $-20°C$ until analysed. They were first screened for absence of or marked reduction in their content of hippuric acid by unidimensional paper chromatography in isopropanol–ammonium hydroxide–water (8:1:1). An aliquot of each urine containing 10 μg of creatinine was applied to the chromatogram. After chromatography, the sheets were first examined under an ultraviolet (UV) light at 254 mμ, and UV-absorbent spots were marked in pencil. The chromatograms were then sprayed with the aroyl glycine reagent (Smith, 1960), and were allowed to dry overnight without heating. With this simple screening test, hippuric acid in normal urine appears as a strong UV-absorbent spot which, after spraying, develops an orange colour characteristic of glycine conjugates of the benzoic acids.

Gas-chromatography

Benzoic acid and hippuric acid were determined quantitatively by a gas chromatographic technique in all urine specimens where preliminary tests had shown a low level of hippuric acid. The urine was acidified with hydrochloric acid to pH 1·0 (pH meter), and was extracted once with a double volume of ethyl acetate, and four more times with equal volumes of ethyl acetate. The combined organic phases were dried overnight over anhydrous sodium sulphate, and the ethyl acetate was removed on a rotary evaporator. The residue was dissolved in methanol-diethyl ether (1:9) and then esterified with diazomethane (Schlenk & Gellerman, 1960). Decanoic acid, 1·0 mg, was added as an internal standard just before the methyl esterification step.

Methyl esters of benzoic and hippuric acid obtained from urine extracts were then determined by gas-chromatography on columns packed with 5 per cent neopentyl glycol adipate on Anakrom SD, 80 to 90 mesh (Analabs, North Haven, Connecticut) on dual column gas-chromatographs equipped with dual flame ionisation detectors. In Vancouver, a MicroTek MT-220 gas-chromatograph was used with 183 $\times$ 0·64 cm i.d. glass columns, while in Norway a Perkin-Elmer 800 gas-chromatograph was used, with stainless steel columns, 200 $\times$ 0·20 cm i.d. The columns were operated at 110°C for 10 minutes after injection of the sample, and their temperature was then raised 10°C/min to a final temperature of 210°C. The amounts of benzoic and hippuric acid present in urine specimens were calculated by measuring the peak areas of their methyl esters on chromatograms with a Technicon integrator-calculator, and comparing them with the areas of the methyl decanoate internal standards. When known amounts of benzoic or hippuric acid were added to normal urines, and the urines were then extracted and analysed as above, recovery rates were 100 per cent for benzoic acid, and 95 to 98 per cent for hippuric acid. Benzoic acid was determined in plasma (first deproteinised by the addition of four volumes of absolute ethanol), and in cerebrospinal fluid, by the same general technique.

Combined gas-chromatography and mass spectrometry for identification of methyl benzoate was performed with a Varian CH 7 mass spectrometer coupled to a Varian 1440 gas-chromatograph, equipped with a single glass column (244 $\times$ 0·20 cm i.d.) packed with 10 per cent OV-17 on Gas-Chrom Q (Applied Science Laboratories, State College, Pennsylvania). Helium was the carrier gas.

Results

Screening for benzoic aciduria

Seventeen of the 307 psychiatric patients showed either a marked reduction or an apparent absence of hippuric acid in their urines when these were screened by paper chromatography. However, only four of these seventeen patients were subsequently shown to excrete benzoic acid in their urine. The remaining thirteen patients excreted low amounts of hippuric acid (0·05 to 0·50 mg/mg of creatinine), but gas-chromatographic analyses of extracts obtained from repeated specimens of their urine failed to reveal any benzoic acid. These false positive screening tests may have been due to low intake of benzoic acid during one or two days prior to the occasions when urine was collected.

Among the 510 control subjects, only one was found whose urine contained benzoic acid. This subject is a 92-year-old woman who, although mentally normal, is bedridden in a nursing home. She has an indwelling catheter and a chronic urinary tract infection, due to a Group D *Streptococcus*. When a small volume of her fresh urine was added to a normal urine, and the latter was incubated overnight at 37°C, much of the hippurate in the normal urine was converted to benzoate. Similar results were obtained by inoculating normal urine with a pure culture of the Group D *Streptococcus* isolated from the urine of this woman. It is obvious that benzoic aciduria in this single mentally normal control subject was the result of hydrolysis of hippuric acid in the urine by a bacterial enzyme. Recently we have encountered a second patient (not included in the control series, because she has arteriosclerotic brain disease) in whom benzoic aciduria was also due to bacterial hydrolysis of hippurate within the urinary tract. This time the hydrolysing organism was a strain of *E. coli*.

Identification of benzoic acid in urine

Fig. 1 shows the very large peak of methyl benzoate, and the absence of a methyl hippurate peak, on the gas-chromatogram of an extract of urine from one of the four psychotic patients with benzoic aciduria. This is contrasted with the absence of methyl benzoate, and the presence of a large methyl hippurate peak, on the gas-chromatogram of an extract of a typical urine sample from a control psychotic patient. The methyl ester of the urinary compound obtained from urine of each of the four benzoate excretors displayed the same retention time as did authentic methyl benzoate during gas chromatography on columns packed with either 5 per cent neopentyl glycol adipate, 20 per cent ethylene glycol adipate, or 10 per cent OV-17.

Urine shown by gas chromatography to contain free benzoate was reduced to pH 3·0 with phosphoric acid, and steam distilled in a Markham still. The distillate was collected, and without the addition of base to trap steam-distillable acids as their non-volatile salts, was reduced to dryness under vacuum on a rotary evaporator at 40°C. The dry powder remaining in the evaporating flask was then sublimed at 12 mm Hg pressure and collected on a cold finger. This purified material, steam-distilled from urine, had the same melting point as did authentic benzoic acid, and did not alter the melting point of benzoic acid when mixed with it. The ultraviolet absorption spectra of the urinary compound and of authentic benzoic acid were similar at neutral, acidic and basic pH. The

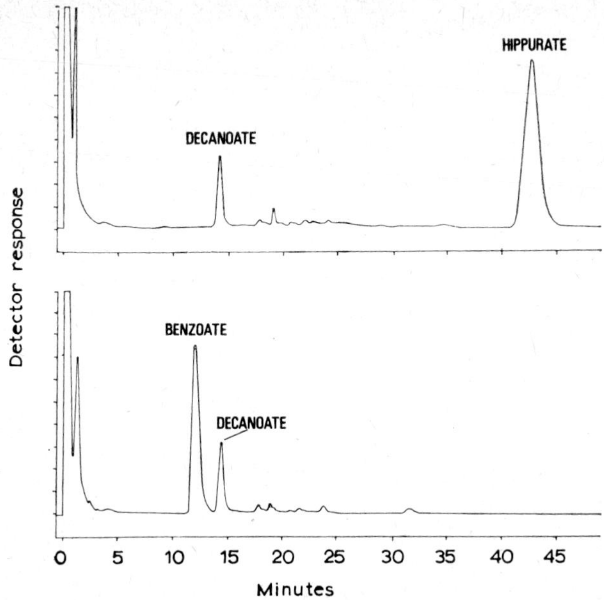

FIG. 1. Gas-chromatogram of methyl esters of urinary acids of a patient with chronic schizophrenia (below) who excreted a large amount of benzoic acid but no hippuric acid, compared to that of another chronic schizophrenic (above) whose urine was normal.

infra-red spectra of the sublimate derived from urine, and of authentic benzoic acid, also were virtually identical.

Finally, identity of benzoic acid was confirmed in a urinary extract from *each* of the four psychotic patients by subjecting the methyl ester preparations to combined gas-chromatography and mass spectrometry. Fig. 2 shows the mass spectrum of the methyl ester of the urinary metabolite, which was identical with that of authentic methyl benzoate. Mass spectrometric analysis revealed a molecular ion at m/e 136. Additional major peaks occurred at m/e 105, compatible with a loss of the OCH_3 group, at m/e 77 representing the benzene ring, and at m/e 50 and 51 representing fragments of the benzene ring.

Benzoate in urines of psychotic patients not an artefact

The benzoic acid found in the urine specimens of the four psychotic patients did not appear to be an artefact due either to the analytical procedures used, or to urinary tract infection. Hippurate in urine was shown not to be hydrolysed during extraction at room temperature, even when the pH of the urine was reduced to values as low as 0·3. It was conceivable that the benzoic acid found in these urines might have

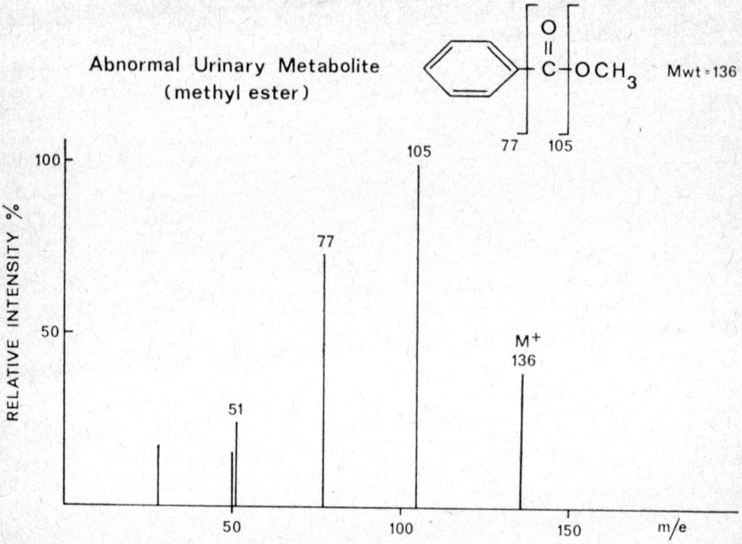

FIG. 2. Mass spectrum of the methyl ester of benzoic acid extracted from the urine of a chronic schizophrenic.

resulted from hydrolysis during the extraction procedure of benzoyl glucuronide, a conjugate of benzoic acid which, under acidic conditions, is likely to be more labile than is hippuric acid. However, direct examination of fresh urines of our four benzoate excretors by a paper-chromatographic technique failed to show any trace of benzoyl glucuronide.

None of the four psychotic benzoate excretors showed any evidence of urinary tract infection on microscopic examination of the urine, and in all four patients benzoic acid disappeared from the urine and reappeared even though the patients were given no antimicrobial drugs. However, facilities were not available to disprove urinary tract infection rigorously by culture techniques. When hippurate was added to the urine of one of the benzoate excretors, and the urine was then incubated at 37°C for 24 hours, there was no increase over the original content of benzoate.

Detailed findings in case 1

Table I shows urinary concentrations of benzoic and hippuric acid found in the urine of case 1 on various occasions during a 5-month period of observation. This patient is a 63-year-old man with chronic schizophrenia who has had a progressive and unremitting psychotic disorder for 38 years, and has been hospitalised for the last 25 years. Initially this patient excreted large amounts of free benzoate, and on some occasions no hippuric acid at all could be detected in his urine. A small amount of benzoic acid (0·57 mg/100 ml) was found in his fasting plasma on the twenty-ninth day of the study period, but benzoic acid was not detectable in his cerebrospinal fluid on that day. The patient was then placed on a special diet which excluded all known sources of benzoic acid for a period of 5 weeks. He continued to excrete some free benzoic acid as late as the eighth day on this diet, but thereafter benzoate was absent and only small amounts of hippurate were found in his urine. After the patient resumed eating a normal diet, only hippurate was found in his urine for several weeks, but later free urinary benzoate reappeared.

Whether the benzoic aciduria temporarily disappeared as a result of the withdrawal of all dietary benzoate, as a result of discontinuing the drugs which the patient had received initially (reserpine and haloperidol) on the sixty-fifth day of the experiment, or for some other reason, could not be determined. However, the eventual reappearance of benzoic aciduria, even though the patient continued to receive no drugs, argues against the possibility that his biochemical abnormality was drug-induced. His ability to conjugate benzoic acid with glycine varied at different times, ranging from none at all to normal amounts. On some occasions, the urinary excretion of benzoate was massive. For instance, if the ratio of benzoic acid to urinary creatinine found in the early morning specimen on day thirty-four (Table I) remained the same throughout a 24-hour period, the

Table I. *Free urinary benzoate in case 1*

Day	*Diet*	*Drugs*	*Benzoic acid* (*mg/mg Creatinine*)	*Hippuric acid* (*mg/mg Creatinine*)
1	Normal	Reserpine & Haloperidol	0·92	0
20	↓	↓	0·66	0
23			0·45	0
32			1·18	0·24
34			1·58	0·11
41	Benzoate-Free			
45	↓		0·21	0
49			0·03	0·13
51			0	0·19
59			0	0·15
65		None		
77	Normal	↓	0	0·45
83	↓		0	1·50
97			0	2·30
104			0·02	0·40
125			0·23	2·27
132			0·17	0·95
139			0·12	2·28

total daily excretion would have been greater than 2 g. No psychiatric or other clinical changes were observed in this patient during the 5-month period of observation. He did not improve mentally during his period of maintenance on a benzoate-free diet, nor did he deteriorate when psychotherapeutic drugs were withdrawn, nor when benzoic aciduria re-appeared after resumption of a normal diet.

Detailed findings in case 2

Table II shows the urinary excretion of benzoic and hippuric acid of case 2 on a number of occasions during 5 months of observation. Also indicated are the changes that occurred in the patient's psychiatric condition during this period. Case 2 is a 64-year-old man with periodic catatonia, who has been described elsewhere by Gjessing (1964). For many years the patient had suffered a long series of episodes of catatonic excitement lasting generally for about 2 weeks, each episode being followed by gradual recovery over a 2- to 3-week period, and then by a 2- to

Table II. *Free urinary benzoate in case 2*

Day	*Drugs*	*Psychotic symptoms* (scale 0 to 4)*	*Benzoic acid* (*mg/mg creatinine*)	*Hippuric acid* (*mg/mg creatinine*)
1	None	2	0·06	0·79
31	↓	2	0·23	0·46
50	↓	2	0·31	0·17
55	Flupenthixol†	1	0	0·22‡
66	↓	1	0	0·50
77	↓	1	0	0·10‡
86	None	3	0·31	0·17
92	↓	3	0·62	0·23
94	↓	2	0·32	0·19
99	↓	2	0·11	0·30
111	↓	1	0	0·69
122	↓	1	0	1·30
125	↓	1	0·24	2·89
127	↓	3	0·41	1·17
129	↓	3	0	0·55
132	↓	2	0	1·13
139	↓	2	0	0·76
150	↓	1	0	1·70

* Psychotic phases commenced abruptly on days 81 and 126.
† Patient received injections of flupenthixol decanoate on days 52 and 67.
‡ Patient briefly on a benzoate-free diet.

k3-wee interval during which his behaviour was virtually normal. His periodic disease had not benefited from numerous electroshock therapies, from treatment with thyroid extract, nor with chlorpromazine. In 1965, he was given reserpine as an antipsychotic drug, and the periodic character of his illness was abolished for a 5-year period. About 6 weeks before the first observation listed in Table II, reserpine therapy was discontinued, and the patient's psychotic symptoms gradually reappeared. These symptoms have been graded on a scale of 0 to 4, 0 representing virtually normal behaviour, and 4 representing the maximum intensity of excitement, sleeplessness, and violence exhibited by this patient during psychotic phases in the earlier years of his illness. As indicated in Table II, the patient showed moderate psychotic symptoms rather steadily during the first 50 days of this study. He then was almost well for about 4 weeks, possibly as a result of having been given two intramuscular injections of flupenthixol, a long-acting thioxanthine tranquilliser. Psychotic phases started abruptly on the eighty-first and the 126th days of the observation period. Each lasted for about 2 weeks, and each was followed by a spontaneous return to near normal psychiatric behaviour.

As in case 1, excretion of free benzoates in the urine of case 2 was intermittent. The highest urinary concentration of benzoic acid observed (on day ninety-two) corresponded to a 24-hour excretion of over 1 g of benzoic acid. On two different occasions, benzoic acid was not detectable in the patient's plasma, but unfortunately these blood specimens were obtained on days when subsequent analyses indicated that the patient was not excreting benzoate. The data in Table II also suggests that this patient's benzoic aciduria was not produced by psychotherapeutic drugs; indeed, benzoate disappeared from his urine when he was given flupenthixol, and reappeared when this drug was stopped.

The most interesting aspect of case 2 was the rough correlation between the presence of free benzoate in the patient's urine and an increase in the severity of his psychotic symptoms. This correlation might have been better documented had it not been for the great difficulty in obtaining any urine specimens from this patient during his psychotic phases, as the result of his threatening behaviour. Observations during the second acute psychotic episode (days 125 to 139 in Table II) indicate that failure to conjugate benzoic acid with glycine preceded the onset of the psychotic phase by at least 24 hours, and that excretion of benzoate in the urine ended before psychiatric improvement was apparent to the physicians and nursing staff.

Other pertinent laboratory findings

The remaining two psychotic patients who excreted benzoic acid were less extensively studied. Benzoic acid was present in the urine of case 3, a 75-year-old man with a depressive psychosis of 4 years duration, on three of four occasions during a 3-month observation period. Case 4, a 68-year-old man with a senile psychosis of 3 years duration, exhibited benzoic aciduria on one of five occasions during a 3-month observation period. The highest concentrations of benzoic acid found in the urine of cases 3 and 4 were 0·39 and 0·25 mg/mg of creatinine respectively.

A battery of standard liver function tests was performed on each of the four benzoic acid excretors, and the normal results made it improbable that gross hepatic failure was responsible for the patients' intermittent failure to conjugate benzoic acid with glycine. In addition, normal values for serum creatinine and blood urea nitrogen in each of the four patients excluded the possibility of severe impairment of renal function. It also seemed unlikely that a deficiency in glycine could account for the benzoic aciduria, since fasting plasma glycine concentrations (measured on an amino acid analyser) were shown to be well within the normal range in each patient at times when the patient's urine contained benzoic acid.

Gas-chromatography of the methyl esters obtained from the four patients' urinary extracts did not reveal any unusual peaks other than methyl benzoate. In addition, hydrolysis of ethyl acetate extracts of the patients' urines in 6 N hydrochloric acid at 110°C for 16 hours did not release any unusual acids from a conjugated form.

DISCUSSION

Our experience suggests that at least 1 per cent of patients hospitalised for chronic psychoses in Norway have benzoic aciduria, and our earlier detection of this abnormality in three chronic schizophrenics in a Canadian mental hospital (Perry *et al.*, 1971) indicates that it occurs in other populations as well. The frequency of benzoic aciduria in mental patients may well be greater than we have found, since the screening test for absence of hippurate would have failed to detect the abnormality in our patients on many occasions. This is clear on inspection of Tables I and II. On some days, these two patients excreted benzoic acid when their urine contained essentially normal amounts of hippuric acid. It is conceivable, of course, that we may have missed some benzoate excretors not only in the mental patients screened, but also among the mentally normal control subjects. Unfortunately one cannot screen for the presence of benzoic acid by means of paper chromatography, in part because of lack of a spray reagent that reacts with benzoic acid to produce a colour, and also because no one solvent system effectively separates benzoic acid from other UV-absorbent or fluorescent compounds in urine.

Why did these four chronically psychotic patients exhibit intermittent benzoic aciduria? The possibility that the benzoic acid arose from hydrolysis of hippurate by bacterial enzymes in the urinary tract, as was the case with the two Canadian subjects described earlier, has not been excluded by careful bacteriological cultures. However, the detection of benzoic acid in the plasma of case 1, and the failure of incubation of fresh urine to increase its content of benzoic acid in case 2, argue against this possibility. There was no reason to believe that an unusually high content of benzoic acid in the hospital diet of our patients could have caused them to excrete unaltered benzoate. Neither did the psychotherapeutic or other drugs the patients received appear to be in any way responsible for the benzoic aciduria. It is also unlikely that defective conjugation of benzoic acid with glycine is simply an enzymatic failure characteristic of ageing in man, since Jellum, Stokke and Eldjarn (1971) have found benzoic acid present in the urine of several children who were classified as severely mentally retarded.

Inability to mobilise glycine for conjugation with benzoyl CoA seems an unlikely explanation for the benzoic aciduria, since concentrations of glycine in fasting plasma were normal. A deficiency in activity of acyl CoA synthetase, the enzyme which converts benzoic acid to benzoyl CoA, also seems improbable. The four Norwegian patients, as well as the three Canadian patients detected earlier, did have increased amounts of acetate in their urine. However, their urine did not contain increased amounts of propionic acid and other volatile fatty acids, and we suspect that the abnormally high amounts of acetic acid found may have come from an unidentified acetate precursor in the urine, rather than having been excreted as acetate itself (Perry *et al.*, 1971). In addition, it seems unlikely that a significant defect in acyl CoA synthetase activity in our patients would have been compatible with their reasonable degree of physical health.

The most likely explanation for the fluctuating benzoic aciduria appears to be an intermittent inhibition of the activity of glycine N-acylase. Since all of the patients on some occasions excreted normal amounts of hippuric acid, and no benzoic acid at all, they probably do not have a genetically-determined defect of the conjugating enzyme itself. The only known inhibitors of glycine N-acylase are ethanol (Amsel & Levy, 1970) and hippurate, the products of the enzymatic reaction (Schachter & Taggart, 1954b). However, none of our patients had access to ethanol, and the amounts of hippurate excreted in their urines were far less than the amounts excreted by other psychotic patients who never excreted free benzoate.

It is conceivable that the glycine conjugate of some unusual organic acid might have acted as an end-product inhibitor of hippurate synthesis in our patients. Glycine N-acylase purified from beef liver mitochondria is known to catalyse the conversion of a number of aliphatic and aromatic acyl thioesters of CoA *in vitro* to the corresponding N-acyl derivatives of glycine (Schachter & Taggart, 1954a). In man, a similar reaction takes place *in vivo* when certain organic acids cannot be further metabolised due to an enzymatic block. Thus large amounts of isovalcryl glycine are excreted in the urine of children with isovaleric acidaemia (Tanaka & Isselbacher, 1967), and β-methylcrotonyl glycine has been found in the urine of patients suffering from another related metabolic disorder of the degradative pathway of leucine (Eldjarn, Jellum, Stokke, Pande & Waaler,

1970). However, we could find no peaks on gas-chromatograms that suggested the presence of a glycine conjugate with a shorter column retention time than that of methyl hippurate. Acid hydrolysates of organic extracts of urines of these patients also revealed no unusual organic acids, and the total amount of glycine recovered in hydrolysates corresponded closely to the amount of hippurate present in the original specimens.

It thus seems most likely that glycine N-acylase was intermittently inhibited in our patients by some metabolite or metabolites as yet unidentified. The fact that the mental illnesses of these four patients had quite different clinical courses, as well as the occurrence of benzoic aciduria among some mentally retarded children, suggests that different inhibitors of benzoic acid conjugation may occur in various clinical conditions.

The correlation between the severity of psychotic symptoms and presence of benzoate in the urine of case 2 suggests a possible causal relationship between benzoic aciduria and mental disorder. It is conceivable that benzoic acid itself has neurotoxic properties. This compound should be relatively lipid-soluble, and it might accumulate in brain tissue when normal conjugation with glycine fails. The fact that case 1 continued to excrete benzoate for 8 days after he had been placed on a benzoate-free diet raises the possibility that appreciable amounts of benzoic acid may have been stored in his lipid tissues. On the other hand, the absence of acute toxic reactions when large loads of sodium benzoate were administered to patients undergoing the Quick test (Quick, 1936), a procedure formerly used to assess impairment of liver function, argues against a direct toxic action of benzoic acid on the brain, at least during acute exposure. Another possibility, of course, is that one or more unknown metabolites which impair the 'detoxification' of benzoic acid to hippuric acid may themselves be neurotoxic and directly produce the mental dysfunction.

The patients with benzoic aciduria in our study may possibly have the same metabolic disorder (or disorders) encountered many years ago by Quastel and Wales (1938, 1940). These investigators found that when they administered sodium benzoate either orally or intravenously to patients with schizophrenia, many of them, especially catatonic schizophrenics, excreted significantly less hippuric acid than did control subjects. At that time, laboratory techniques for detecting and measuring benzoic acid in urine were not available.

Conclusions

Benzoic aciduria occurs in at least 1 per cent of hospitalised adults with chronic psychoses, and does not appear to be caused by diet, psychotherapeutic drugs, liver disease, or other factors related to prolonged hospitalisation. The abnormality may possibly be due to inhibition of the conjugation of benzoic acid with glycine by one or more unknown metabolites, and either benzoic acid or the latter might play a part in producing mental dysfunction. Since certain strains of bacteria that cause chronic urinary tract infection can hydrolyse hippuric acid in the urine to free benzoic acid, care must be taken when further cases of benzoic aciduria are discovered to exclude such artefactual causes of benzoic-aciduria by careful bacteriological studies.

Acknowledgements

We thank Dr Leiv R. Gjessing for generously making his laboratory available for this study, and for his help with the patients. Dr Egil Jellum of Oslo kindly performed the mass spectrometric analyses, and Dr R. H. Wright of Vancouver performed the infra red spectral analyses. We also thank Mr L. Gibson for culture and identification of urinary organisms, and Drs L. Lesk, M. Hestrin and A. Trites for helping in obtaining urine samples from normal subjects. The following persons gave useful technical assistance: O. Borud, A Frenningsmoen, P. Gjesdahl. M. Kloster, R. Langseth and T. L. Perry, Jnr. This work was supported by grants from the Medical Research Council of Canada, the British Columbia Medical Services Foundation and the National Institute of Mental Health.

REFERENCES

AMSEL, L. P. & LEVY, G. (1970) *Proc. Soc. exp. Biol.* (*N.Y.*), **135**, 813.

ARMSTRONG, M. D. (1963) *In* Lyman, F. L. (ed.) *Phenylketonuria.* Springfield: Charles C. Thomas, p. 81.

ELDJARN, L., JELLUM, E., STOKKE, O., PANDE, H. & WAALER, P. E. (1970) *Lancet*, **ii**, 521.

FURIA, T. E. (1968) *C.R.C. Handbook of Food Additives.* Cleveland: The Chemical Rubber Co., p. 143.

GJESSING, L. R. (1964) *J. psychiat. Res.*, **2**, 123.

JELLUM, E., STOKKE, O. & ELDJARN, L. (1971) *Scand. J. clin. Lab. Invest.*, **27**, 273.

PERRY, T. L., HANSEN, S., DIAMOND, S., MELANÇON, S. B. & LESK, D. (1971) *Clin. chim. Acta*, **31**, 181.

QUASTEL, J. H. & WALES, W. T. (1938) *Lancet*, **ii**, 301.

QUASTEL, J. H. & WALES, W. T. (1940) *Lancet*, **i**, 402.

QUICK, A. J. (1936) *Arch. int. Med.*, **57**, 544.

SCHACHTER, D. & TAGGART, J. V. (1954a) *J. biol. Chem.*, **208**, 263.

SCHACHTER, D. & TAGGART, J. V. (1954b) *J. biol. Chem.*, **211**, 271.

SCHLENK, H. & GELLERMAN, J. L. (1960) *Ann. Chem.*, **32**, 1412.

SMITH, I. (1960) *In Chromatographic and Electrophoretic Techniques* 2nd edn., Vol. 1. London: William Heinemann, p. 291.

TANAKA, K. & ISSELBACHER, K. J. (1967) *J. biol. Chem.*, **242**, 2966.

DISCUSSION
(of the Paper by Dr Perry)

Gompertz (*London*). There was a report of trans-methylhexenoic acid being present in the sweat of chronic schizophrenics. Could this be a candidate for an acyl compound inhibiting glycine N-acylase?

Perry (*Vancouver*). I think it highly unlikely that trans-3-methyl-2-hexenoic acid could be an inhibitor of glycine N-acylase in our patients. On reading that this acid had been detected in the sweat of patients with chronic schizophrenia (Smith, K., Thompson, G. F. & Koster, H. D., 1969, *Science*, **166**, 398), my colleagues and I searched for it in the sweat of eleven patients with schizophrenia who had an unusual odour. We could not detect trans-3-methyl-2-hexenoic acid in the sweat of any of these patients, but instead found that artefacts with identical gas-chromatographic behaviour were dissolved from the polyethylene bags used to collect the sweat, and were also present in the diethyl ether used for extraction of the sweat (Perry, T. L., Melançon, S. B., Lesk, D. & Hansen, S., 1970, *Clin. chim. Acta*, **30**, 721). I am not convinced that this compound is present in the sweat of chronic schizophrenics.

Seakins (*London*). Dr Perry, did you do any loading tests with either benzoic or quinic acids on the patients with benzoic aciduria? Since quinic acid is an important precursor of benzoic acid, were the diets also free of quinic acid?

The delay in the cessation of benzoic acid excretion when this acid and its precursors were removed from the diet suggests the large bowel as a source of benzoic acid. Were these patients constipated? Was there any diurnal variation in the excretion of benzoic acid?

Perry. The benzoic acid-free diet given in case 1 also excluded quinic acid. Loads of sodium benzoate were given to cases 1 and 2, with recovery of part of each load as benzoate and part as hippurate. However these loading tests provided no additional information beyond that found with the natural loading provided by a general diet. It is likely that our patients may have been constipated; chronically hospitalised psychotic patients often are. We did not explore the possibility of a diurnal variation in the excretion of benzoic acid. All urine specimens analysed were first morning specimens.

Carson (*Belfast*). Were any CSF studies carried out?

Perry. CSF was examined for benzoic acid in case 1 on a single occasion. None could be detected.

PYROGLUTAMIC ACIDURIA. A NEW INBORN ERROR OF METABOLISM POSSIBLY IN THE "γ-GLUTAMYL CYCLE" PROPOSED FOR AMINO ACID TRANSPORT

by

LORENTZ ELDJARN, ODDVAR STOKKE
AND EGIL JELLUM

WE have recently described a new inborn error of metabolism characterised by the excretion in the urine of 25–40 g per 24 hours of L-pyroglutamic acid (pyrrolidonecarboxylic acid, Fig. 1). The patient was a 19-year-old male, whose parents are not consanguineous. Neither in the urine of the patient's brother and parents nor in twenty-three close relatives (nephews, uncles and aunts) could we demonstrate pyroglutamic acid (Jellum *et al.*, 1970; Eldjarn *et al.*, 1972).

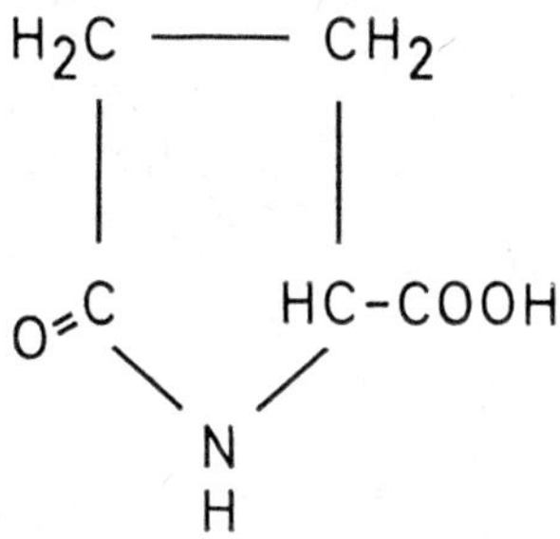

Pyroglutamic acid
(Pyrrolidone-2-carboxylic acid)

FIG. 1.

The patient is of normal height and weight. He shows symptoms of spastic tetraparesis and cerebellar disturbances with intention tremor and atactic gait and increased resistance to passive movements. Voluntary movements are retarded, with pronounced tremor and impaired co-ordination. For years he has suffered from periods of vomiting and sporadic haematemesis. Possibly related to this, a diaphragmatic hernia developed (Kluge *et al.*, 1971). After surgical treatment a persistent metabolic acidosis precipitated the discovery of his inborn error of metabolism. Despite early symptoms of retarded psychomotor development, he attended elementary school up until the age of 14 years after which he stayed for 3 years in a special school for mentally retarded children. His IQ level as determined by the Wechsler test is approximately 60.

Thus, we are faced with a new inborn error of metabolism with mental retardation and signs of organic neurological disturbances. The excretion of formidable amounts of cyclised glutamic acid raises a number of questions related to the significance of glutamic acid, glutamine and γ-aminobutyric acid in the metabolism of the central nervous system. As a start, however, we have found it necessary to investigate the biochemical significance of pyroglutamic acid, which is known to occur in minor amounts in the γ-chain of immunoglobulins (Putnam & Kohler, 1969) and in thyroid-stimulating hormone-release factor (Nair *et al.*, 1970). Small amounts have also been found in human urine following severe burns (Tham, Nystrøm & Holmstedt, 1968). The formidable amounts which our patient excretes raises the puzzling problem whether pyroglutamic acid is a hitherto overlooked key metabolite in the nitrogen metabolism of mammals.

Is Pyroglutamic Acid Production Related to the Cyclic Process of Urea Synthesis?

During the 18 months we have observed the patient, he excreted on an ordinary diet approximately 50 per cent of his urinary nitrogen in the form of pyroglutamic acid, whereas urea is correspondingly reduced. At first it was therefore considered a possibility that due to a disturbance in the normal urea production, pyroglutamic acid might occur as a side product. Its close chemical relationship to glutamic acid might indicate a block in the formation of 'free ammonia' from glutamic acid by glutamic acid dehydrogenase. 'Free ammonia' in activated form (carbamyl phosphate) contributes 50 per cent of the urea nitrogen whereas the other half stems from the amino acid pool by way of aspartic acid and argininosuccinic acid (Fig. 2).

The possible relationship between pyroglutamic acid production and urea synthesis was tested in several ways. Firstly, the patient was given large doses of NH_4HCO_3 (0·42 moles in the course of 4 days). The excess nitrogen was completely recovered in the form of urea and urinary ammonia, whereas the pyroglutamic acid excretion remained unchanged. Thus, the conversion of ammonium ions to urea proceeds normally, independent of the pyroglutamic acid production. Secondly the protein intake of the patient was varied from 120 g to 20 g per 24 hours (in the latter case in the form of essential amino acids only). This resulted in a concomitant variation in the excretion of urea (from 0·3 to 0·02 moles per 24 hours). In contrast, pyroglutamic acid remained nearly constant during this treatment. When minor variations did occur there appeared to be a certain parallelism between pyroglutamic acid and NH_4^+ excretion.

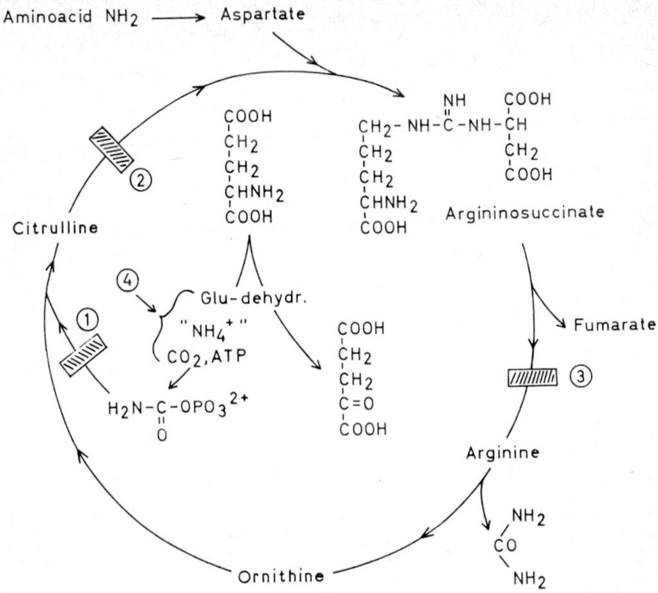

FIG. 2. The cyclic process of urea synthesis. Inborn errors are previously described at (1) = hyperammonaemia; (2) = citrullinaemia; and (3) = argininosuccinic aciduria. It appears unlikely that the metabolic error in pyroglutamic aciduria is to be found at (4).

Both these experiments show that drastic variations in the gross intake and catabolism of nitrogen result in corresponding changes in urea production whereas no clear effect on pyroglutamic acid production occurs. In particular, no indication of a defective 'free ammonia' production could be shown. Thus, it is unlikely that the pyroglutamic acid excretion is caused by a disturbance in the urea production.

Is pyroglutamic Acid Formation Related to Ammonium Ion Production in the Kidneys?

In our patient the urinary clearance for pyroglutamic acid is at least five times that of creatinine, a finding which indicates that pyroglutamic acid may be produced in the kidneys. The high clearance values follow from the fact that small amounts of pyroglutamic acid only are found in his serum (less than 5 mg per 100 ml).

In the above protein feeding experiments it was consistently seen that the urinary excretion of pyroglutamic acid and of ammonium ions vary in parallel, the former being approximately twice the latter on a molar basis. It is generally accepted that the γ-amide of glutamine is the major source of urinary ammonia. We therefore considered that pyroglutamic acid and

NH_4^+ production in the kidneys might stem from glutamine by an abnormal behaviour of the ammonium producing enzyme system. To study this possibility, the acid base status of the patient was significantly altered. On an ordinary diet the patient presents with a chronic metabolic acidosis with a base excess from -4 to -8 meq/l. After the administration of excessive amounts of $NaHCO_3$ for a period of three days, a metabolic alkalosis occurred with blood pH of 7·45 and base excess of $+4$ meq/l. However, the urine remained acidic (pH 5). A slight drop in the NH_4^+ production was seen, whereas pyroglutamic acid excretion remained essentially unchanged. Similar findings were recorded when the $NaHCO_3$-induced metabolic alkalosis was maintained for several weeks.

An attempt was also made to influence the pyroglutamic acid production by a peroral load of L-glutamine (0·17 mmoles = 25 g) distributed over 24 hours. The excretion of pyroglutamic acid and NH_4^+ remained essentially unaltered, whereas the greater part of the glutamine-N was recovered as urea.

Our experimental data therefore do not support the idea that pyroglutamic acid stems from the ammonium ion producing system of the kidneys. The 'paradoxical' aciduria with unchanged NH_4^+ production despite metabolic alkalosis may be ascribed to the fact that the pyroglutamic acid excretion also remained unchanged (pyroglutamic acid has a $pK_a \approx 3$).

Is Pyroglutamic Acid Production Related to the Renal Handling of Amino Acids?

Up till now we have found only one experimental condition which significantly alters the excretion of pyroglutamic acid in our patient. When the serum level of amino acids was trebled over a period of 3 hours by intravenous infusion of a mixture of synthetic L-amino acids, the amounts of pyroglutamic acid excreted per hour was simultaneously increased by a factor of 2–3. This finding makes it reasonable to correlate the pyroglutamic acid formation with the recently described 'γ-glutamyl cycle' (Orlowski & Meister, 1970). It is assumed that the ultra-filtered free amino acids at the apical end of the tubular cells are converted to γ-glutamyl dipeptides in a reaction with glutathione and a transpeptidase. The dipeptides serve as intracellular transport form of the amino acids which in turn is liberated into the blood stream by a γ-glutamyl cyclotransferase (γ-glutamyl lactamase) with the concomitant production of pyroglutamic acid from the γ-glutamyl residue. The pyroglutamic acid is postulated to be converted to glutamic acid by some unknown enzyme system (Fig. 3).

Our findings may be a strong indication that the ideas of the 'γ-glutamyl cycle' are essentially correct. It should be recalled that per 24 hours approximately 35 g of free amino acids are ultrafiltered in the

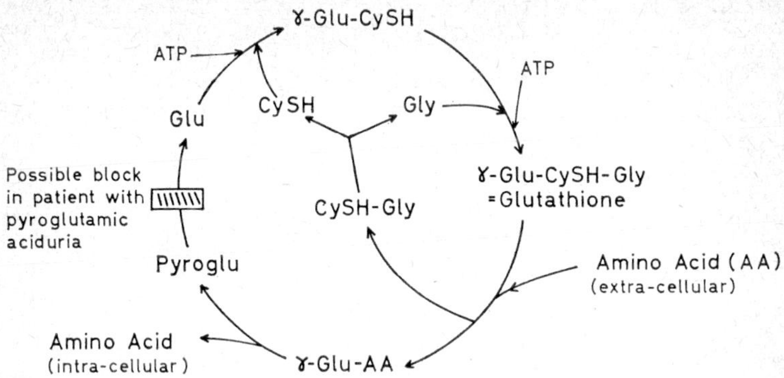

FIG. 3. The gammaglutamyl cycle as proposed by Orlowski and Meister (1970) for the tubular reabsorption of amino acids by the kidneys.

kidneys. The above hypothesis pre-supposes an equimolar formation of pyroglutamic acid in the course of tubular reabsorption. Thus, the amounts of pyroglutamic acid found in our patient correspond fairly well with those expected. On the other hand, it is rather unexpected that such a defect in the amino acid reabsorption system should be without consequences for the amino acids in the urine: the amino acid excretion pattern in our patient is within normal limits.

The Enzyme Defect in Our Patient

A likely explanation for the fact that our patient excretes formidable amounts of pyroglutamic acid would thus be that the compound is a normal intermediate in the mammalian metabolism and that the patient has a defect in some enzyme system which removes pyroglutamic acid (e.g. converts it to glutamic acid). In a number of experiments we have collected data which strongly support this interpretation. Thus, normal controls convert i.v. injected [U-^{14}C] L-pyroglutamic acid rapid to respiratory CO_2 (17 per cent of the dose in the course of 2½ hours), whereas unchanged pyroglutamic acid could not be recovered from the urine. This oxidation rate corresponds with that of glutamic acid. In the patient, on the other hand, the conversion of [U-^{14}C] pyroglutamic acid to respiratory CO_2 takes place at a very low rate, only 1·7 per cent being expired in 2½hours. In addition, the patient excretes unchanged labelled pyroglutamic acid in the urine, 30 per cent and 66 per cent being recovered after 2½ and 24 hours, respectively. A slow conversion to glutamic acid obviously also takes place, since a total of 12·5 per cent of injected dose could be recovered in this form in the urine after 24 hours.

Attempts were also made to study the precursor relationship of urinary pyroglutamic acid in our patient. Following the i.v. injection of U-^{14}C-glutamic acid, labelled pyroglutamic acid slowly appeared in the urine, with its maximum after 1½ hours. At this time, the specific activity of urinary pyroglutamic acid was found to be only 1/100 of that of serum glutamic acid. Also the i.v. injection of ^{14}C pyruvate gives rise to labelled pyroglutamic acid with a maximum in specific activity after approximately 2 hours. These findings indicate that glutamic acid as such is not the immediate precursor of urinary pyroglutamic acid. It should be recalled that ordinary diet contains only approximately 10 g per day of glutamic acid whereas our patient excretes about 35 g of pyroglutamic acid per 24 hours. Whatever the immediate precursor of pyroglutamic acid, the carbon atoms of its 'glutamic acid residue' must for the larger part stem from the tricarboxylic acid cycle.

Fractionation by thin layer chromatography of the urinary radioactivity in the above tracer experiments revealed in addition to labelled pyroglutamic and glutamic acid, also a slower-moving component. The specific activity of this compound was at the maximum in the first urinary sample following the injection of labelled compound as against pyroglutamic and glutamic acid with a maximum after 1½–2 hours. Upon acid hydrolysis of the unknown compound followed by thin layer chromatography, the radioactive band co-chromatographed with glutamic acid. Also in the serum of the patient is found an unknown compound which upon hydrolysis gives rise to glutamic acid. It is considered likely that these unknown compounds may be identical, possibly the dipeptide or dipeptides which may be the immediate precursor of pyroglutamic acid.

Conclusion

The discovery of a patient with an enzyme defect closely related to the metabolism of glutamic acid, demonstrating mental retardation and signs of organic neurological disturbances may offer a unique opportunity to study the significance of glutamic acid, glutamine and γ-amino butyric acid for the function of the central nervous system. In the present publication we have given data which strongly indicate that pyroglutamic acid should not be looked upon as the result of some side reaction of nitrogen metabolism. On the contrary, our patient seems to be deficient in some enzyme system which normally removes pyroglutamic acid (possibly by a conversion to glutamic acid). Thus, pyroglutamic acid most probably should be considered a key metabolite in the nitrogen metabolism of mammals, possibly involved in amino acid transport mechanisms.

References

Eldjarn, L., Jellum, E. & Stokke, O. (1972) Clin. chim. Acta, in the press.

Jellum, E., Kluge, T., Børresen, H. C., Stokke, O. & Eldjarn, L. (1970) *Scand. J. clin. Lab. Invest.*, **26**, 327.

KLUGE, T., BØRRESEN, H. C., JELLUM, E., STOKKE, O., ELDJARN, L. & FRETHEIM, B. (1972) *Surgery*, **71**, 104.
NAIR, R. M. G., BARRETT, J. F., BOWERS, C. Y. & SCHALLY, A. V. (1970) *Biochemistry*, **9**, 1103.
ORLOWSKI, M. & MEISTER, A. (1970) *Proc. nat. Acad. Sci.* (Wash.), **67**, 1248.
PUTMAN, F. W. & KOHLER, H. (1969) *Naturwissenschaften*, **56**, 439.
THAM, R., NYSTRØM, L. & HOLMSTEDT, B. (1968) *Biochem. Pharmacol.*, **17**, 1735.

DISCUSSION
(of the Paper by Professor Eldjarn)

Watts (*Harrow*). Can Dr Eldjarn explain why there is no aminoaciduria at all in this patient?

Eldjarn (*Oslo*). We have given much thought to this problem. What we can say at the present stage is only that according to the Orlowski-Meister reabsorption mechanism, the process of amino acid reabsorption is already accomplished before the postulated action of the enzyme which is defective in our patient.

Nyhan (*La Jolla*). We have shown (*Cancer Res.*, **18**, 385, 1958) that glutamate is a source of pyroglutamic acid *in vivo* in rat kidney but in no other organs. Thus we were interested in Meister's hypothesis on the methyl-γ-glutamyl cycle and its role in transport. This patient offers an exciting chance to test the hypothesis. Have you tested individual amino acids to see which of them participate in this transport system?

Eldjarn. The mixture of the synthetic L-amino acids which we used ('Vamine' Astra AB, Sweden) contains a total of eighteen different L-amino acids. Our experiment does therefore not permit any conclusions concerning the absorption of specific amino acids.

Cusworth (*London*). If the postulated mechanism of amino acid transport in the kidney exists it is almost certain that the γ-glutamyl dipeptide will not be 100 per cent reabsorbed—a very small amount at least will leak into the urine. In 1955 Dr Westall (*Biochem. J.*, **60**, 247) isolated the amino acids from 100 l of his own urine and found small peptides. The 10 or so γ-glutamyl di-peptides might well be amongst them.

If there is a pyroglutamate to glutamate block in this patient there may well be a pile-up of the γ-glutamyl dipeptide. As Dr Watts has suggested one would anticipate an increased amino acid excretion here, but if the effect is only a small increase in these dipeptides this might not be detected by ordinary amino acid studies, using paper, thin layer or ion-exchange chromatograms. Maybe one needs to collect 100 l of urine and isolate the amino acids and small peptides. It may then be found that there is a significant increase in the γ-glutamyl dipeptides.

Eldjarn. Of course it is our working hypothesis that gamma-glutamyl dipeptides may be the substance of the 'glutamine X' which appears as a rapid labelled compound in the urine of the patient after the injection of [^{14}C]-glutamate, -pyruvate and -glutamine. It is our intention to attempt isolation and structural determination of 'glutamine X' by more sophisticated means so that the collection of a hundred litres of urine can be avoided.

PRIMARY HYPEROXALURIA

by

R. W. E. WATTS

PRIMARY hyperoxaluria was first defined on the basis of the association of recurrent calcium oxalate urinary calculi, and a continuous greatly increased urinary excretion of oxalate (Archer, Dormer, Scowen & Watts, 1957a). Post-mortem studies showed widespread deposits of calcium oxalate particularly in the kidneys, the tunica media of small muscular arteries, the myocardium, the rete testis and in growing bones (Scowen, Stansfeld & Watts, 1959). Similar post-mortem findings had been described previously in cases where the urinary excretion had not been measured (Chou & Donohue, 1952; Burke, Baggenstoss, Owen, Power & Lohr, 1955; Neustein, Stevenson & Krainer, 1955; Dunn, 1955; Lund & Reske-Nielsen, 1956; Hollosi, 1957; De Toni, Durand & Rosso, 1957). Most of the cases present in childhood and die in adolescence or in early adult life. A few of the patients either die in infancy or present as adults with urinary calculi, and the urinary oxalate excretion should be measured in all cases of calcium oxalate urinary stones. The simple method described by Archer, Dormer, Scowen and Watts (1957b) is suitable for diagnosis and screening purposes, but more elaborate methods are needed if the significance of relatively small changes in the urinary oxalate excretion is to be assessed. Gibbs and Watts (1969) used an isotope dilution method of analysis and found that the urinary oxalate excretion increases during childhood, adult values being reached between the ages of 12 and 14 years. The effect of age was largely abolished if the results were related to a standard body surface area. Hockaday, Frederick, Clayton and Smith (1965) used an isotope dilution method of analysis which involved a different method of isolating and purifying the urinary oxalate, and obtained virtually identical results. They quote extreme ranges of between 10 and 56 mg of anhydrous oxalic acid/24 hours/1·73 m^2 for children younger than 14 years, and 18–47 mg of anhydrous oxalic acid/24 hours/1·73 m^2 for adults; the corresponding values obtained by Gibbs and Watts (1969) were 28–56 and 21–52 mg/24 hours/1·73 m^2 respectively.

Cases of primary hyperoxaluria have recently been subclassified as type I in which hyperglycollic aciduria also occurs, and type II in which the urinary excretion of $L(+)$glyceric acid is also increased, the urinary glycollate excretion being normal (Smith & Williams, 1967; Williams & Smith, 1967). Both types follow a similar clinical course.

The genetic data are compatible with the disease being due to the operation of a rare autosomal recessive gene (Archer, Dormer, Scowen & Watts 1958a; Scowen, Watts & Hall, 1959), although there is some evidence that it may follow a dominant pattern of inheritance in some families (Shepard, Lee & Krebs, 1960). There have been no genetic studies which have taken account of the recent subdivision of primary hyperoxaluria into types I and II.

Oxalate does not appear to have an intermediary metabolic role in man and animals (Weinhouse & Friedman, 1951; Curtin & King, 1955; Brubacher, Just, Bodur & Bernhard, 1956; Elder & Wyngaarden, 1960) and the metabolic pathways which lead to oxalate are shown in Fig. 1. Dean, Watts and Westwick (1968) presented evidence for the incorporation of the carbon skeleton of glycine into oxalate by two alternative metabolic pathways in intact man. Both of the possible intermediates of the 2-oxoglutarate:glyoxylate carboligase reaction which were proposed by Schlossberg, Richert, Bloom and Westerfeld (1968) are shown, the hypothetical regeneration of 2-oxoglutarate being indicated by the dotted arrow; the second molecule of CO_2 is eliminated non-enzymatically. The dynamics of the incorporation of the C_1 carbon atom of ascorbic acid into urinary oxalate was studied by Atkins, Dean, Griffin and Watts (1964) and Atkins, Dean, Griffin, Scowen and Watts (1965). Other metabolic pathways join the cycle at points A and B.

Cattell, Spencer, Taylor and Watts (1962) found [^{14}C]oxalate to be excreted by a combination of glomerular filtration and active tubular secretion, and that there was evidence for some passive back-diffusion of oxalate from the renal tubule. Zarembski and Hodgkinson (1963) reported a large net tubular reabsorption of oxalate in normal and hyperoxaluric human subjects, however Williams and Smith (1971) have recently obtained results in man using [^{14}C]oxalate which agree with those of Cattell *et al.* (1961).

Attempts to identify the metabolic abnormality which underlies primary hyperoxaluria at the enzyme level have been complicated by lack of previous knowledge of the normal biochemical reactions which glyoxylate undergoes in man. Three different metabolic lesions have been reported on the basis of studies using isolated tissue preparations. These are: (1) reduced activity of the soluble glyoxylate:2-oxoglutarate carboligase (Fig. 1) in type I primary hyperoxaluria, the corresponding mitochondrial enzyme being normal (Koch, Stokstad, Williams & Smith 1967); (2) reduced *D*-glyceric dehydrogenase activity in type II primary hyperoxaluria (Broyer & Berger, 1968; Williams & Smith, 1968); (3) reduced metabolism of glyoxylate to CO_2 and glycine in kidney tissue from two sibs; however, these patients were studied before the sub-types of primary hyperoxaluria were recognised (Dean, Watts & Westwick, 1966), and other workers have suggested that the reduced transaminase activity may

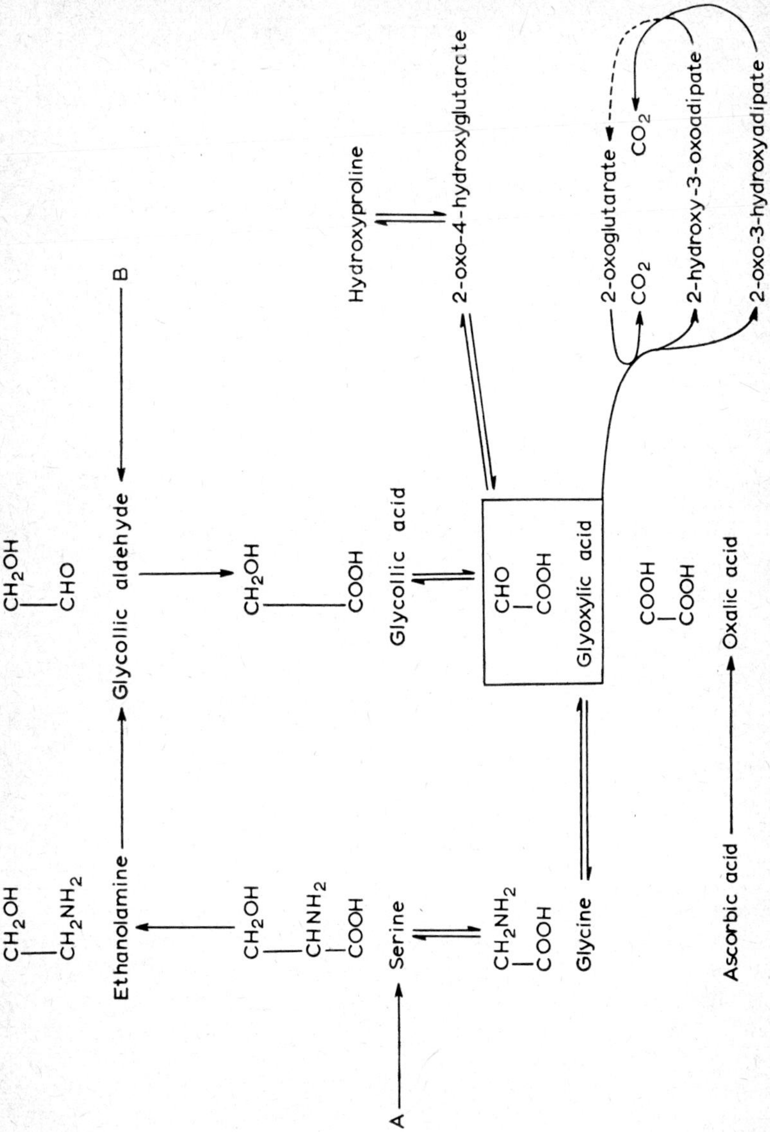

FIG. 1. The metabolic pathways which lead to oxalate.

not be peculiar to primary hyperoxaluria (Williams, Wilson & Smith, 1967). Metabolic lesions (1) and (2) would be expected to impair the metabolism of glyoxylate and make more of this compound available for oxidation to oxalate (Fig. 1). Such a mechanism would be compatible with the results of the earlier *in vivo* studies of the incorporation of the labelled carbon atom of [1—^{13}C]glycine into oxalate which suggested that the primary abnormality in the disease involved a failure to metabolise glyoxylate normally by other, at the time unidentified, metabolic pathways (Crawhall, Scowen & Watts, 1958; 1959). It is also in accord with the reported reduced conversion of [1—^{14}C]glyoxylate and [1—^{14}C]glycollate to expired $^{14}CO_2$ and urinary [1—^{14}C]glycine with increased incorporation of the isotope into urinary oxalate and glycollate *in vivo* (Frederick, Rabkin, Richie & Smith, 1963; Hockaday, Clayton & Smith, 1965).

The enzyme glyoxylate:2-oxoglutarate carboligase catalyses the synergistic decarboxylation of glyoxylate and 2-oxoglutarate which was described in liver mitochondria by Crawhall and Watts (1962a,b). Koch *et al* (1967) suggested that two such isoenzymes exist, the mitochondrial one referred to above which has normal activity in primary hyperoxaluria, and an isoenzyme which occurs in the soluble fraction of several tissues. The latter is deficient in type I primary hyperoxaluria, the accumulated glyoxylate being either oxidised to oxalate or reduced to glycollate (Koch *et al.*, 1967). Williams and Smith (1968; 1971) explain the association of *L*(+)glyceric aciduria, hyperoxaluria and *D*-glyceric acid dehydrogenase deficiency in type II primary hyperoxaluria by assuming that hydroxypyruvate accumulates, and is reduced to *L*-glycerate by an $NADH_2$ requiring enzyme. They then suggest that the NAD which is generated promotes the oxidation of glyoxylate to oxalate. These authors were able to show that hydroxypyruvate had the effect on oxalate production from glyoxylate which their theory predicted in human erythrocytes and leucocytes, rat liver and with a commercial preparation of beef heart lactate dehydrogenase. However, they present no evidence for the assertion upon which the theory is based, namely that hydroxypyruvate accumulates in type II primary hyperoxaluria, nor do they present any evidence for the identity of the enzymes which are concerned *in vivo*. (*See note added in proof.*)

Attempts to reduce the urinary excretion of oxalate in primary hyperoxaluria by protein restriction have been unsuccessful (Gibbs & Watts, 1967). Similarly, although the administration of large doses of sodium benzoate in order to deplete the precursor glycine pool produces an evanescent reduction in the urinary oxalate excretion (Archer, Dormer, Scowen & Watts, 1958b), this is not of any therapeutic value. Attempts to inhibit oxalate formation by the use of drugs which inhibit one of the enzymes which are known to be capable of catalysing the oxidation of aldehydes to carboxylic acids have likewise been unrewarding. The drugs used were allopurinol to block xanthine:oxygen oxidoreductase (EC 1.2.3.2) (Gibbs & Watts, 1968), calcium carbimide (Solomons, Goodman & Riley, 1967; Zarembski, Hodgkinson & Cochran, 1967; Gibbs & Watts, 1968; King, 1970), disulfiram (Gibbs & Watts, 1968) to block aldehyde: NAD oxidoreductase (EC 1.2.1.3), and acetomenaphthone to block aldehyde:oxygen oxidoreductase (EC 1.2.3.1) (Gibbs & Watts, 1968). These studies were made in the absence of any precise knowledge of the enzymes which catalyse the oxidation of glyoxylate to oxalate in the disease and the most recent work (Gibbs, 1971) shows that the main enzyme catalysing this reaction in the soluble fraction of human liver is lactate:NAD oxidoreductase (EC 1.1.1.27). Only a minor part of the enzyme activity of the tissue with respect to the oxidation of glyoxylate to oxalate in the soluble fraction of human liver tissue could be accounted for by xanthine:oxygen oxidoreductase (EC 1.2.3.2) and glycollate oxidase (EC 1.1.3.1).

Dent and Stamp (1970) recommend the administration of sufficient magnesium hydroxide to increase the urinary excretion of magnesium and thereby inhibit calcium oxalate precipitation in the urine. They consider that this has materially improved the prognosis in nine children with the disease. Methylene blue, in common with other dyes, inhibits crystal growth *in vitro*. It is excreted in the urine and has been recommended for trial in the treatment of primary hyperoxaluria (Sutor, 1969; 1970).

Large oral doses of pyridoxine (for example 450 mg of pyridoxine hydrochloride daily in divided doses) reduce the urinary oxalate excretion to levels which are intermediate between the pre-treatment and normal ranges of values in some patients (Gibbs & Watts, 1969; 1970). The administration of both pyridoxine and magnesium oxide simultaneously appears to have a less clear-cut effect on the urinary oxalate excretion than pyridoxine alone. It is also logical to reduce the urinary calcium excretion, and the possible importance of this has been emphasised by recent work on the physical chemistry of stone formation (Hodgkinson & Nordin, 1971; Robertson, Peacock & Nordin, 1971).

Renal transplantation cannot be recommended in these cases because calcium oxalate deposits form in the grafted kidney (Deodhar, Tung, Zuhlke & Nakamato, 1969). The oxalate ion can be removed from the body by peritoneal dialysis and by haemodialysis. The latter method of treatment was tried intensively in one case by Cattell and Watts (1970) and although the blood urea level and other parameters of renal function responded in the anticipated manner, the patient died having developed ischaemic skin lesions on her digits and heart block (Coltart & Hudson, 1971). The usual post-mortem picture of disseminated oxalosis was present in this case.

Note added in proof. Evidence has now been obtained for the role of lactate: NAD^+ oxidoreductase (lactate dehydrogenase) in the oxidation of glyoxylate to oxalate in the human heart as well as in the liver. (Gibbs & Watts, submitted for publication); and in blood cells (Smith, Bauer & Williams, 1971, *J. Lab. clin. Med.*, **78,** 245.)

REFERENCES

ARCHER, H. E., DORMER, A. E., SCOWEN, E. F. & WATTS, R. W. E. (1957a) *Lancet*, **ii**, 320.

ARCHER, H. E., DORMER, A. E. SCOWEN, E. F. & WATTS, R. W. E. (1957b) *Clin. Sci.*, **16**, 405.

ARCHER, H. E., DORMER, A. E., SCOWEN, E. F. & WATTS, R. W. E. (1958a) *Ann. hum. Genet.*, **22**, 373.

ARCHER, H. E., DORMER, A. E., SCOWEN, E. F. & WATTS, R. W. E. (1958b) *Brit. med. J.*, **i**, 175.

ATKINS, G. L. DEAN, BETTY M., GRIFFIN, WENDY J. & WATTS, R. W.E. (1964) *J. biol. Chem.*, **239**, 2975.

ATKINS, G. L., DEAN, BETTY M., GRIFFIN, WENDY J. & WATTS, R. W. E. (1965) *Clin. Sci.*, **29**, 305.

BROYER, M. & BERGER, R. (1968) *Presse med.*, **76**, 2395.

BRUBACHER, G., JUST, M., BODUR, H. & BERNHARD, K. (1956) *Ztschr. Physiol. Chem.*, **304**, 173.

BURKE, C. E., BAGGENSTOSS, A. H., OWEN, C. A., POWER, M. H. & LOHR, O. W. (1955) *Pediatrics*, **15**, 383.

CATTELL, W. R., SPENCER, A. G., TAYLOR, G. W., WATTS, R. W. E. (1962) *Clin. Sci.*, **22**, 43.

CATTELL, W. R. & WATTS, R. W. E. (1970) Unpublished data.

CHOU, L. Y. & DONOHUE, W. L. (1952) *Pediatrics*, **10**, 660.

COLTART, D. J. & HUDSON, R. E. B. (1971) *Brit. Heart. J.*, **33**, 315.

CRAWHALL, J. C., SCOWEN, E. F. & WATTS, R. W. E. (1959) *Lancet*, **ii**. 806.

CRAWHALL, J. C. & WATTS, R. W. E. (1962a) *Biochem. J.*, **85**, 163.

CRAWHALL, J. C. & WATTS, R. W. E. (1962b) *Clin. Sci.*, **23**, 163.

CURTIN, C. O. 'H. & KING, G. C. (1955) *J. biol. Chem.*, **216**, 539.

DE TONI, G., DURAND, P. & ROSSO, C., (1957) *Minerva pediat.*, **IX**, 23.

DEAN, BETTY M., WATTS, R. W. E. & WESTWICK, WENDY J., (1966) *Biochem. J.*, **105**, 701.

DEAN, BETTY M., WATTS, R. W. E. & WESTWICK, WENDY J. (1968) *Clin. Sci.*, **35**, 325.

DENT, C. E. & STAMP, T. C. B. (1970) *Arch. Dis. Childh.*, **43**, 313.

DEODHAR, S. D., TUNG, K. S. K., ZUHLKE, V. & NAKAMOTO, S. (1969) *Arch. Path.*, **87**, 118.

DUNN, H. G., (1955) *Amer. J. Dis. Child.*, **90**, 58.

ELDER, T. D. & WYNGAARDEN, J. B. (1960) *J. clin. Invest.*, **39**, 1337.

FREDERICK, ELIZABETH, W., RABKIN, M. T., RICHIE, R. H., SMITH, L. H. (1963) *New Engl. J. Med.*, **269**, 822.

GIBBS, DOROTHY A., (1971) Clin Sci., **41**, 30; and unpublished data.

GIBBS, DOROTHY A. & WATTS, R. W. E. (1967) *Arch. Dis. Childh.*, **42**, 505.

GIBBS, DOROTHY A., & WATTS, R. W. E. (1968) *Arch. Dis. Childh.*, **43**, 313.

GIBBS, DOROTHY A. & WATTS, R. W. E. (1969) *J. Lab. clin. Med.*, **73**, 901.

GIBBS, DOROTHY A., & WATTS, R. W. E. (1970) *Clin. Sci.*, **38**, 277.

HOCKADAY, T. D. R., FREDERICK, E. W., CLAYTON, J. E. & SMITH, L. H. (1965) *J. Lab. clin. Med.*, **65**, 677.

HOCKADAY, T. D. R., CLAYTON, J. E. & SMITH, L. H. (1965) *Arch. Dis. Childh.*, **40**, 485.

HODGKINSON, A. & NORDIN, B. E. C. (1971) *Biochem. J.*, **122**, 5*P*.

HOLLOSI, KATHERINE, (1957) *Zbl. allg. Path. path. Anat.*, **96**, 220.

KING, J. S. (1970) *Invest. Urol.*, **8**, 1.

KOCH, J., STOKSTAD, E. L. R., WILLIAMS, H. E. & SMITH, L. H. (1967) *Proc. nat. Acad. Sci.*, **57**, 1123.

LUND, T. & RESKE-NIELSEN, EDITH, (1956) *Acta path. microbiol. scand.*, **38**, 353.

NEUSTEIN, H. B., STEVENSON, S. S., KRAINER, L. (1955) *J. Pediat.*, **47**, 624.

ROBERTSON, W. G., PEACOCK, M. & NORDIN, B. E. C. (1971) *Clin. Sci.*, **40**, 365.

SCHLOSSBERG, M. A., BLOOM, R. J., RICHERT, D. A. & WESTERFELD, W. W. (1968) *Biochemistry*, **7**, 333.

SCOWEN, E. F., STANSFELD, A. G. & WATTS, R. W. E. (1959) *J. Path. Bact.*, **77**, 195.

SCOWEN, E. F. WATTS, R. W. E. & HALL, E. G. (1959) *Ann. hum. Genet.*, **23**, 367.
SHEPARD, T. H., LEE, L. W., & KREBS, E. G. (1960) *Pediatrics*, **25**, 869.
SMITH, L. H. & WILLIAMS, H. E. (1967) *In* Nyhan, W. L. (ed.) *Amino acid metabolism and genetic variation*. New York: McGraw-Hill.
SOLOMONS, C. C., GOODMAN, S. I. & RILEY, C. M. (1967) *New Engl. J. Med.*, **276**, 207.
SUTOR, J. (1969) *Brit. J. Urol.*, **51**, 171.
SUTOR, J. (1970) *Brit. J. Urol.*, **42**, 389.
WEINHOUSE, S. & FRIEDMAN, B., (1951) *J. biol. Chem.*, **191**, 707.
WILLIAMS, H. E., & SMITH, L. H. (1967) *In* Nyhan, W. L. (ed.) *Amino Acid metabolism and genetic variation*. New York: McGraw-Hill.
WILLIAMS, H. E. & SMITH, L. H. (1968) *New Engl. J. Med.*, **278**, 233.
WILLIAMS, H. E. & SMITH, L. H. (1971) *Clin. Sci.*, **41**, 213.
WILLIAMS, H. E., WILSON, MARGARET & SMITH, L. H. (1969) *J. Lab. clin. Med.*, **70**, 494.
ZAREMBSKI, P. M. & HODGKINSON, A. (1963) *Invest. Urol.*, **1**, 87.
ZAREMBSKI, P. M., HODGKINSON, A. & CHOCHRAN, M. (1967) *New Engl. J. Med.*, **277**, 1000.

PHYSICAL CHEMISTRY OF CALCIUM OXALATE CRYSTALLISATION

by

A. HODGKINSON, R. W. MARSHALL AND W. G. ROBERTSON

THE two principal forms of calcium oxalate occurring in nature are the monohydrate, whewellite, and the dihydrate, weddellite. Both forms occur widely in fossil rocks, in plant and animal tissues and in urinary tract calculi but the monohydrate is generally the more common type. The monohydrate is monoclinic in crystallisation whereas the dihydrate is tetragonal but both hydrates crystallise in a great variety of forms. The crystals are usually very small, making it difficult to perform structural analyses by X-ray diffraction methods but Cocco and Sabelli succeeded in determining the lattice parameters of whewellite in 1962 and their findings were confirmed in studies of large needle-shaped crystals from the desert plant, Yucca rupicola by Arnott, Pautard and Steinfink (1965).

The structure of the tetragonal dihydrate was determined by Sterling (1965) who also resolved earlier uncertainties regarding the exact water content of this hydrate. The structure proposed by Sterling requires a basic hydrate content of 2 moles of water per mole of calcium with additional 'zeolitic' water up to 0·5 mole per mole of calcium. A tri-hydrate has also been described (Hammarsten, 1927, 1956; Lecomte, Pobequin & Wyart, 1945) but this has not been fully characterised.

Both solubility and instability increase with increasing water of crystallisation, the tri-hydrate being about three times more soluble than the monohydrate (Hammarsten, 1956) (Table I). An excess of calcium ions, such as occurs in urine, favours the formation of the less stable higher hydrates which are then thought to lose some of their water of crystallisation to form the monohydrate (Tovborg-Jensen, 1941; Hammarsten, 1956). However, the conditions which favour the formation of the different hydrates are still only poorly understood, (Lyon & Vermeulen, 1965).

Table I. *The hydrates of calcium oxalate* (Hammarsten, 1956)

	Solubility M × 10^5)		*Solubility Product* (K^{0}_{sp})	
	(25°C)	(37°C)	(25°C)	(37°C)
Ca $(COO)_2$. $1H_2O$	4·40	5·50	8·96	8·79
Ca $(COO)_2$. $2H_2O$	7·65	9·50	8·57	8·44
Ca $(COO)_2$. $3H_2O$	13·30	16·40	8·22	8·10

Crystallisation requires some degree of supersaturation of the solution with respect to an appropriate solid phase and this is determined by comparing the ionic activity product with the known solubility and formation products of the relevant salt (Fig. 1). Solutions having activity

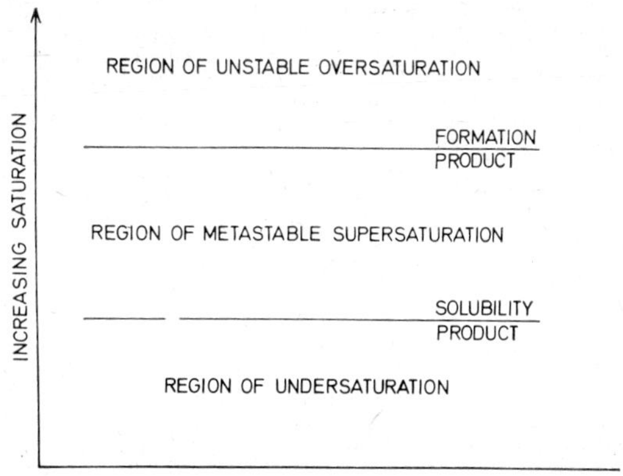

FIG. 1. The three states of saturation of aqueous solutions.

products below the solubility product are said to be 'undersaturated' and any crystals of the salt which are present, will tend to dissolve. Above the solubility product there is a region of 'metastable supersaturation' in which a solution can exist for relatively long periods without crystallisation occurring but crystallisation can be induced by the addition of a suitable nucleus. Above the formation product, spontaneous nucleation can occur and crystal growth is usually rapid.

Until recently it was not possible to measure calcium oxalate activity products in biological fluids accurately because of the difficulty in measuring calcium and oxalate ion activities, as distinct from their total concentrations, but specific liquid and solid state electrodes are now available which are capable of measuring calcium ion activities with an acceptable degree of accuracy (Ross, 1967; Schultz, Petersen, Mask & Buck, 1968). Oxalate ion activities cannot be measured directly at present but can be calculated from the pH and ionic strength of the solution and the stability constants of the relevant complexes (Robertson, 1969).

The steps involved in the calculation of ionic activity products are summarised in Fig. 2. The ionic strength (μ) is calculated from the equation

$$\mu = \tfrac{1}{2}\Sigma\, C_i\, Z_i^2$$

where C_i is the concentration of the ion and Z_i the charge on the ion.

The ionic strength is then used to calculate the activity coefficient, which is a measure of the extent to which the solution departs from ideal

CALCULATION OF ACTIVITY PRODUCTS

ACTIVITY PRODUCT $(K^{o}) = \{C^{+}\} \times \{A^{-}\}$

$$= [C^{+}] \times f_{c} \times [A^{-}] \times f_{a}$$

ACTIVITY COEFFICIENT :

$$-\log f_{i} = \frac{A\, Z_{i}^{2}\sqrt{\mu}}{1 + B_{a}^{o}\sqrt{\mu}} \quad \text{(Debye and Huckel 1923)}$$

$$-\log f_{i}^{\pm} = 0.5\, z_{1} z_{2} \left\{ \frac{\sqrt{\mu}}{1 + \mu} - 0.3\,\mu \right\} \quad \text{(I}$$

IONIC STRENGTH $(\mu) = \frac{1}{2}\sum C_{i}\, Z_{i}^{2}$

FIG. 2. Formulae used in the calculation of activity products (see text for details).

behaviour. This may be calculated from some form of the Debye-Huckel equation, such as that proposed by Davies (1938, 1962).

$$-\log f\pm = 0{\cdot}5\, Z_1\, Z_2 \left\{ \frac{\sqrt{\mu}}{1+\sqrt{\mu}} - 0{\cdot}3\mu \right\}$$

where $f\pm$ is the mean ionic activity coefficient and Z_1, Z_2 are the valencies of the constituent ions. That this equation accurately predicts activity coefficients at the ionic strength in plasma and urine is shown in Fig. 3. in which calcium ion activity coefficients, calculated by the Davies equation, are compared with measured values obtained with the Orion calcium electrode (Orion Research Inc. Cambridge, Mass.).

Finally, the activity coefficient is used to calculate the activity product K^{o} from the equation:

$$K^{o} = [C^{+}] \times f_{c} \times [A^{-}] \times f_{a}$$

where the brackets represent the concentrations of anions and cations and f_a, f_c are the activity coefficients.

So far, most studies of activity products in biological fluids have been confined to urine. Using the techniques described above, Robertson, Peacock and Nordin (1968) found that normal urine is generally in a state of metastable supersaturation with respect to calcium oxalate. Subsequent studies of diurnal variations in activity products have shown that normal urine may be oversaturated with respect to calcium oxalate for short periods of the day and during these periods calcium oxalate crystals will

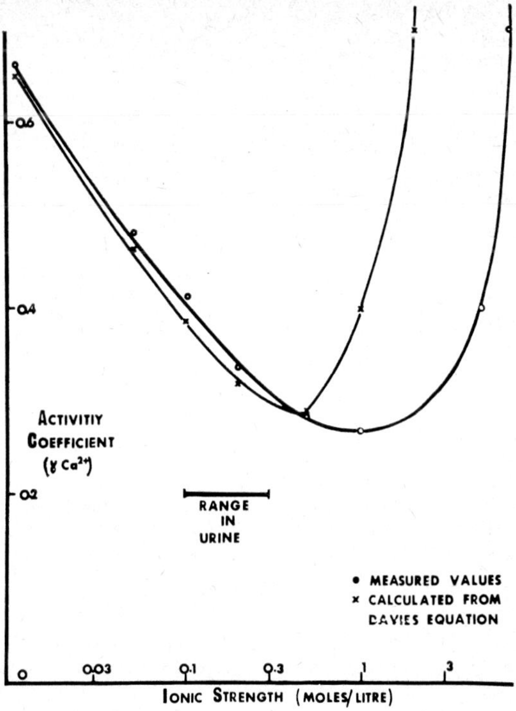

FIG. 3. Comparison of calcium ion activity coefficients. o, measured with the Orion calcium electrode; x, calculated from the equation of Davies (1938).

form spontaneously. Such periods of oversaturation are more frequent and pronounced in patients with idiopathic calcium oxalate renal stones, due mainly to an increased concentration of calcium ions in the urine. Even more pronounced periods of oversaturation occur in primary hyperoxaluria, due mainly to the increased concentration of oxalate ions (Robertson, Peacock & Nordin, 1968; Hodgkinson, Marshall & Cochran, 1971).

The degree of saturation of blood with respect to calcium oxalate can only be assessed in general terms at present because of uncertainties regarding the exact concentration of oxalic acid in plasma. Improvements in analytical techniques during the past 30 years have led to a progressive lowering of the normal range in man and the most recent chemical and enzymic methods indicate values ranging from 50 to 150 μg per 100 ml (Hodgkinson & Zarembski, 1968; Knowles & Hodgkinson, 1971). Still lower values ranging from 3 to 45 μg per 100 ml have been obtained by using isotope dilution analysis (Elder & Wyngaarden, 1960; Williams & Smith, 1968).

Approximately half of the oxalic acid in normal plasma appears to be ionised, the remainder being complexed with calcium and to a lesser extent with magnesium (Table II). Ultrafiltration studies indicate that

Table II. *The state of oxalic acid in plasma*

	K(37°C)	Per cent of total§
Ca Ox	$7{\cdot}07 \times 10^{3}$*	44·0
Mg Ox	$2{\cdot}57 \times 10^{3}$†	7·0
H Ox-	$2{\cdot}10 \times 10^{4}$‡	0·1
Oxalate ion (Ox^{2-})		49·0
	Total =	100·0

* Gelles, E. & Salama, A. (1958).
† Pederson, K. J. (1939).
‡ Pinching, G. D. & Bates, G. (1948).
§ I = 0·15; pH = 7·4.

little or no oxalate is bound to plasma proteins at physiological pH (Cattell, Spencer, Taylor & Watts, 1962; Zarembski & Hodgkinson, 1965).

These observations suggest that plasma is normally undersaturated with respect to all three hydrates of calcium oxalate but supersaturation probably occurs in uraemia when the plasma oxalate level may be increased several times (Zarembski, Hodgkinson & Parsons 1966; Knowles & Hodgkinson, 1972) (Fig. 4). This probably accounts for the frequent occurrence of calcium oxalate crystals in renal tissue in patients dying from renal failure (Fanger & Esparza, 1964).

Other conditions associated with raised plasma oxalate levels and the deposition of calcium oxalate crystals in renal and other tissues are oxalate poisoning (Zarembski & Hodgkinson, 1967), ethylene glycol poisoning (Bove, 1966) and methoxyflurane poisoning (Frascino, Vanamee & Rosen, 1970). Plasma oxalate levels appear to be normal in patients with primary hyperoxaluria except in the terminal oliguric phase (Crawhall & Watts, 1961; Zarembski & Hodgkinson, 1963).

Oxalic acid concentrations in most tissues are low (Scowen, Stansfeld & Watts, 1959; Wyngaarden & Elder, 1966; Hodgkinson & Zarembski, 1968) but the kidney appears to be a notable exception in having a steep oxalate concentration gradient between the cortex and inner medulla (Wright & Hodgkinson, 1971). In the rat, the concentration of oxalic acid at the tip of the renal papilla averaged 1·8 mmol per kg wet weight of tissue, compared with 0·38 in the cortex and 0·11 in urine (Fig. 5). Previous studies in a number of mammalian species, including man, have shown that the renal papilla also contains high concentrations of calcium,

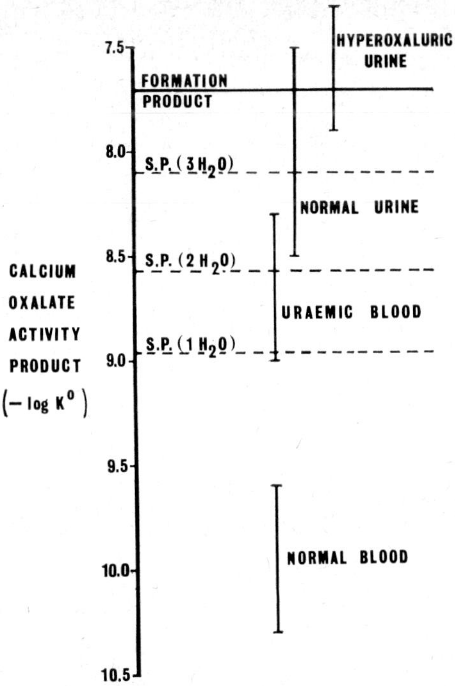

FIG. 4. Approximate ranges of calcium oxalate activity products in normal and uraemic blood compared with the ranges in normal and hyperoxaluric urine.

relative to other tissues (Gains, Michaels, Thwaites & Trounce, 1968; Cooke, 1971). If all the calcium and oxalic acid in the renal papilla were freely ionised then the ion product would be approximately 2×10^{-5}. While the ionic strength and activity coefficients in such a medium are unknown it is clear that this product is many times the formation product and that much of the calcium and oxalic acid in the normal papilla must be bound or compartmented in such a way that it cannot precipitate.

In conclusion, it appears that the risk of calcium oxalate precipitation in the blood and most other body fluids and tissues is small since they are normally undersaturated with respect to calcium oxalate. However, supersaturation may occur in renal failure and this can be relieved by haemodialysis (Zarembski, Rosen & Hodgkinson, 1969). In contrast, the urinary tract is normally exposed to considerable risk from calcium oxalate precipitation since high concentrations of calcium and oxalic acid occur in the renal papilla, and urine is commonly supersaturated or even oversaturated with respect to calcium oxalate. Recent measures to prevent

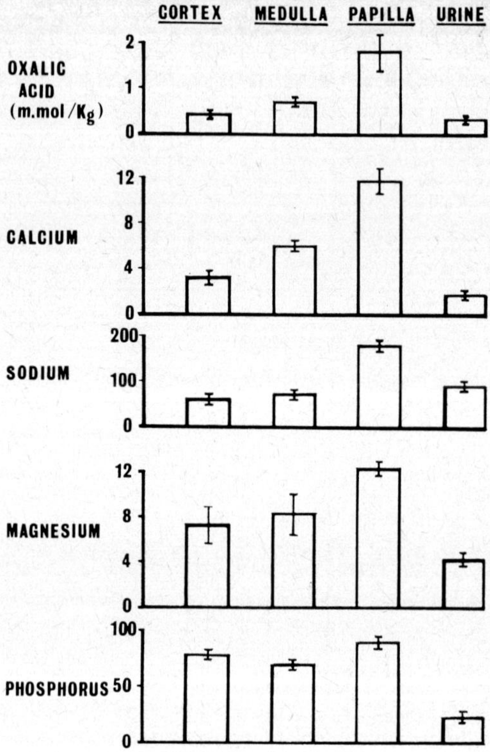

FIG. 5. Solute concentrations in the renal cortex, medulla and papilla compared with those in urine of the normal rat. The vertical lines denote ±I.S.E. (n = 27).

calcium oxalate crystallisation in calcium stone formers, particularly those with the inborn error of primary hyperoxaluria, include the oral administration of magnesium (Dent & Stamp, 1970; Melnick, Landes, Hoffman & Burch, 1971) pyridoxine (Gibbs & Watts, 1970) and methylene blue (Boyce, McKinney, Long & Drach, 1967; Sutor, 1970) but none of these treatments has been finally proven yet.

REFERENCES

ARNOTT, H. J., PAUTARD, F. G. E. & STEINFINK, H. (1965) *Nature*, **208**, 1179.

BOVE, K. E. (1966) *Amer. J. clin. Path.*, **45**, 46.

BOYCE, W. H., MCKINNEY, W. M., LONG, T. T. & DRACH, G. W. (1967) *J. Urol.*, **97**, 783.

CATTELL, W. R., SPENCER, A. G., TAYLOR, G. W. & WATTS, R. W. E. (1962) *Clin. Sci.*, **22**, 43.

COCCO, G. & SABELLI, C. (1962) *Proc. Verbali Mem, series A*, **69**, 289.

COOKE, S. A. R. (1971) *Brit. J. Urol.*, **43**, 130.

CRAWHALL, J. C. & WATTS, R. W. E. (1961) *Clin. Sci.*, **20**, 357.

DAVIES, C. W. (1938) *J. chem. Soc.*, 2093.
DAVIES, C. W. (1962) *Ion association*. London: Butterworth.
DENT, C. E. & STAMP, T. C. B. (1970) *Arch Dis. Childh.*, **45**, 735.
ELDER, T. D. & WYNGAARDEN, J. B. (1960) *J. clin. Invest.*, **39**, 1337.
FANGER, H. & ESPARZA, A. (1964) *Amer. J. clin. Path.*, **41**, 597.
FRASCINO, J. A., VANAMEE, P. & ROSEN, P. P. (1970) *New Eng. J. Med.*, **283**, 676.
GAINS, N. A., MICHAELS, C. W., THWAITES, M. Z. & TROUNCE, J. R. (1968) *Nephron*, **5**, 352.
GELLES, E. & SALAMA, A. (1958) *J. chem. Soc.*, 3683.
GIBBS, D. A. & WATTS, R. W. E. (1970) *Clin. Sci.*, **38**, 277.
HAMMARSTEN, G. (1927) *C. R. Lab. Carlsberg*, **17**, 1.
HAMMARSTEN, G. (1956) *In* Butt, A. J. (ed.), *Etiologic Factors in Renal Lithiasis*. Springfield: Chas. C. Thomas, p. 89.
HODGKINSON, A., MARSHALL, R. W. & COCHRAN, M. (1971) *Israel J. Med. Sci.*, in press.
HODGKINSON, A. & ZAREMBSKI, P. M. (1968) *Calc. Tiss. Res.*, **2**, 115.
KNOWLES, C. F. & HODGKINSON, A. (1972) *Analyst*, in the press.
LECOMTE, J., POBEQUIN, T. & WYART, J. (1945) *J. Phys. Radium* (Paris), **6**, 22.
LYON, E. S. & VERMEULEN, C. W. (1965) *Invest. Urol.*, **3**, 309.
MELNICK, I., LANDES, R. R., HOFFMANN, A. A. & BURCH, J. F. (1971) *J. Urol.*, **105**, 119.
PEDERSON, K. J. (1939) *Trans. Faraday Soc.*, **35**, 277.
PINCHING, G. D. & BATES, G. (1948) *J. Res. nat. Bur. Stand.*, **40**, 405.
ROBERTSON, W. G. (1969) *Clin. chim. Acta*, **24**, 149.
ROBERTSON, W. G., PEACOCK, M. & NORDIN, B. E. C. (1968) *Clin. Sci.*, **34**, 579.
ROSS, J. W. (1967) *Science*, **156**, 1378.
SCHULTZ, F. A., PETERSEN, A. J., MASK, C. A. & BUCK, R. P. (1968) *Science*, **162**, 267.
SCOWEN, E. F., STANSFELD, A. G. & WATTS, R. W. E. (1959) *J. Path Bact.*, **77**, 195.
STERLING, C. (1965) *Acta cryst.*, **18**, 917.
SUTOR, D. J. (1970) *Brit. J. Urol.*, **42**, 389.
TOVBORG-JENSEN, A. (1941) *Acta chir. scand.*, **85**, 473.
WILLIAMS, H. E. & SMITH, L. H. (1968) *Amer. J. Med.*, **45**, 715.
WRIGHT, R. J. & HODGKINSON, A. (1971) *Invest. Urol.*, **9**, 369.
WYNGAARDEN, J. B. & ELDER, T. D. (1966) *In* Stanbury, J. B. etc. (eds.), *The Metabolic Basis of Inherited Disease*. New York: McGraw-Hill, p. 189.
ZAREMBSKI, P. M. & HODGKINSON, A. (1963) *Invest Urol.*, **1**, 87.
ZAREMBSKI, P. M. & HODGKINSON, A. (1965) *Biochem. J.*, **96**, 717.
ZAREMBSKI, P. M. & HODGKINSON, A. (1967) *J. clin Path.*, **20**, 283.
ZAREMBSKI, P. M., HODGKINSON, A. & PARSONS, F. M. (1966) *Nature*, **212**, 511.
ZAREMBSKI, P. M., ROSEN, S. M. & HODGKINSON, A. (1969) *Brit. J. Urol.*, **41**, 530.

DISCUSSION
(of Papers by Dr Watts and Dr Hodgkinson)

Cusworth (*London*). Is the blood oxalate level significantly raised in primary hyperoxaluria and is the oxalate decarboxylase method of measurement a possible way of identifying patients with primary hyperoxaluria?

Hodgkinson (*Leeds*). Accurate measurement of the low concentration of oxalic acid in blood still presents technical difficulties. On present evidence it would appear that plasma oxalate levels are not appreciably raised in patients with primary hyperoxaluria, until renal function becomes grossly impaired, when very high concentrations up to 3 or 4 mg per 100 ml can occur.

With regaıd to the identification of patients with primary hyperoxaluria this is readily achieved by measuring the oxalic acid in the urine by conventional chemical methods. The oxalate decarboxylase method of measurement may offer marginal advantages because of the specificity of the enzyme but it might be more useful to determine the excretion of glyoxylic, glycollic and glyceric acids in order to distinguish between primary hyperoxaluria types I and II (Williams and Smith, 1968).

Watts (*Harrow*). Dr Hodgkinson, how well do calculated and measured values of ion activities agree in these complicated systems?

Hodgkinson. Dr Roberston, in our department, has shown that calculated and measured values of calcium ion activities agree well in at least two complex systems, namely, human plasma ultrafiltrates and urine (Robertson, Peacock & Nordin, 1968; Robertson, 1969).

Curtius (*Zurich*). What is the role of urinary peptides in inhibiting stone formation?

Hodgkinson. It has been known for many years that hypertrophic cartilage from rachitic rats will mineralise *in vitro* when incubated in serum or appropriate solutions. Thomas and Howard showed in 1959 that mineralisation did not occur in normal urine, despite the presence of high concentrations of calcium and phosphorous, but it occurred in urine from many patients with renal stones. This difference was attributed to an inhibitor of mineralisation which was present in normal urine and absent or inactive in stone-forming urine. Subsequent studies led to the isolation of two low molecular weight peptides with high inhibitory activity (Howard, Thomas, Barker, Smith & Wadkins, 1967, *Johns Hopkins med. J.*, **120**, 119). However, we were unable to demonstrate any significant difference in the activities of these peptides when isolated from normal and stone-forming urines (Robertson, Hambleton & Hodgkinson, 1969, *Clin. chim. Acta*, **25**, 247). I understand that Howard and his colleagues now believe these peptides to be contaminants, the inhibitory activity being due to some other unidentified molecule.

THE SEMI-QUANTITATIVE ESTIMATION OF α-KETO ACIDS IN THE CLINICAL LABORATORY

by

PETER LUTZ, GERHARD MICHAEL VON REUTERN AND ROLF-PETER WILLIGMANN

BETWEEN 10 and 15 keto acids may occur in human plasma and urine; most of them have the carbonyl group in the α-position to the carboxyl group. This chemical configuration is rather sensitive to heat; CO_2 may be split off, and an aldehyde will be formed. Thus, gas liquid chromatography (GLC) will give rise to problems, and thin layer chromatography (TLC) may retain an important role in the detection of these compounds.

Carbonyl groups are highly reactive; numerous addition reactions often followed by elimination reactions occur, e.g. (Fig. 1) with hydrazine,

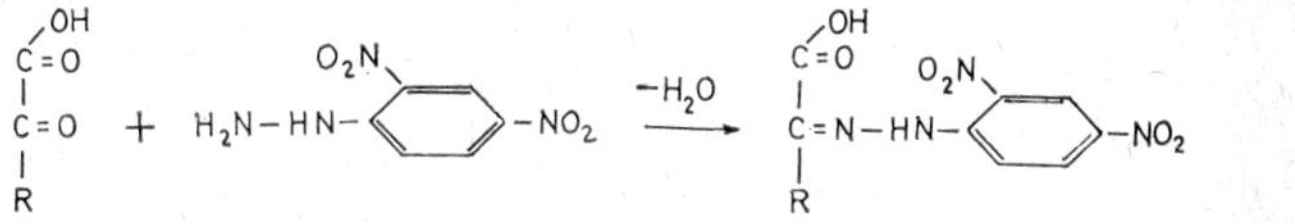

FIG. 1. The reaction of α-ketoacids with 2,4-dinitrophenylhydrazine.

phenylhydrazine, and 2,4-dinitrophenylhydrazine resulting in hydrazones, in the example given in 2,4-dinitrophenylhydrazones (2,4-DNPH). From the analyst's viewpoint these compounds are superior to others in being well-defined crystalline deep-yellow substances; one can dispense with any staining technique after the chromatographic separation. But there are difficulties, too: hydrazones in solution form two isomers; possibly the strongly acidic hydrogen at the nitrogen atom will form a hydrogen bond to the carbonyl group of the carboxyl group and thus stabilise a six-membered ring; apparently an equilibrium exists between this form and the form with the ring split, that is as drawn in Fig. 1. Fortunately, one form strongly predominates; possibly a single isomer might be formed if the hydrogen atom were substituted by a methyl group; but a 2,4-dinitrophenylhydrazine modified in such a way is not commercially available, and therefore investigations are lacking.

Our method does not claim to be very original in using 2,4-dinitrophenylhydrazine, as many authors have done so before us (see Table I). Only Ronakainen used methyl esters, and Menkes converted the hydrazones into the corresponding amino acids by hydrogenation; since the chromatographic detection of amino acids is a well-established

Table I. *Survey of separation methods for alpha-ketoacids*

Author	*Derivative used*	*Technique (PC, TLC, Eph)*	*Number of Sep. Acids*	*Remarks*
D. Cavallini *et al.* (1949)	2,4-DNPH	PC, 1-dimensional	2	
H. Kaeser *et al.* (1959)	,,	,,	7	
J. H. Menkes (1960)	2,4-DNPH Aminoacids	,,	7	
J. Dancis *et al.* (1963)	2,4-DNPH	TLC, 1-dimensional	6	
P. Ronkainen (1966)	2,4-DNPH, methyl ester	TLC, 1-dimensional, silicagel, activated	7	
,, (1967)	2,4-DNPH	TLC, 1-dimensional, silicagel, neutral	7	
J. Cotte *et al.* (1967)	,,	TLC, 1-dimensional, silicagel		
P. Smith (1967)	2·4-DNPH	PC, 1-dimensional	24	R_F values close to each other
A. S. Saini (1967)	,,	PC descending run	4	
R. F. Coward *et al.* (1969)	,,	PC, 2-dimensional	7	
,, (1968)	,,	PC, 1-dimensional		for PKU and tyrosyluria
H. H. Berlet (1968)	,,	TLC, 2-dimensional, silicagel	6	
H.-J. Stan *et al.* (1969)	,,	TLC, 1-dimensional, silicagel	6	
P. Lutz *et al.* (1969)	,,	TLC, 2-dimensional, silicagel	10	
H. Bayzer (1971)	,,	TLEph + TLC, cellulose	4	

method, the identification of the corresponding keto acids may become easier; but for routine analysis, catalytic hydrogenation is tedious. A shift to TLC instead of paper chromatography (PC) might be noticed from Table I, analogous to the trend in the chromatography of amino acids, and silicagel is preferred; the 2-dimensional technique is useful if more than 6 keto acid hydrazones must be separated.

Table II shows in schematic form the preparation of the samples: at first, urine creatinine is estimated as a reference substance; it is difficult to get 24 hours urine collections from infants, therefore a reference must be chosen with which the keto acid excretion can be compared. In the first step, 20 ml of urine are mixed with 10 ml of the strongly acidic dinitrophenylhydrazine solution; if the urine sample contains a large amount of keto acids, the hydrazones will precipitate at once, otherwise the yellow colour will deepen during 4 hours. The following extraction elutes the hydrazones out of the watery phase, the next one separates acidic from neutral hydrazones, and the third extraction removes cations

Table II. *The detection of ketoacids in urine*

Preceding steps: (1) estimation of creatinine
(2) screening for ketoacids: if total amount is elevated: TLC

Procedure: 20 ml of urine + 10 ml of 2,4-dinitrophenylhydrazine solution (0·2 per cent in 2N HCl)

↓

Reaction during 4 hours at room temperature, mixture protected against light

↓

Extraction with 3 × 20 ml of di-isopropylether, organic phases are combined

↓

Extraction of ether solution with 6 × 10 ml of sodium bicarbonate solution (0·2 per cent in water)

↓

Extraction of water solution with 10 ml of ethylacetate

↓

Adjustment to pH 1 by addition of 1N HCl

↓

Extraction of water solution with 3 × 10 ml of ethylacetate

↓

Evaporation to dryness of the organic phase

↓

Residue is taken up in 0·5–1·0 ml of ethylacetate according to the creatinine concentration.

↓

TLC : Silicagel plates (MERCK), 10 × 10 or 20 × 20 cm, are charged with an aliquot of the ethylacetate solution corresponding to 0·15 mg creatinine;
solvent 1st dimension : acetone/iso-amylalcohol/water 50:50:1 (v/v)
solvent 2nd dimension : (a) iso-amylalcohol/0·25N ammonium hydroxide 20:1 (v/v) (b) chloroform/glacial acetic acid 100:7(v/v), twice!

from the acidic hydrazones. We tried to use ion exchange resins instead of extraction with solvents; but the poor solubility of the hydrazones makes this type of separation difficult.

In TLC, silicagel proved to be superior to cellulose, but the R_F values may differ considerably unless standardised plates are used. As solvents, the combination of acetone/*iso*-amylalcohol/water in the vertical and of *iso*-amylalcohol/ammonium hydroxide, followed by chloroform/glacial acetic acid in the horizontal direction proved best; the spots are distributed evenly all over the plate. Most of the isomeric forms assemble in one spot (Fig. 2, spot 5) and thus do not complicate the interpretation of the chromatographic picture. The separation of the spots 1–3 can be improved by raising the water percentage in the vertical direction solvent.

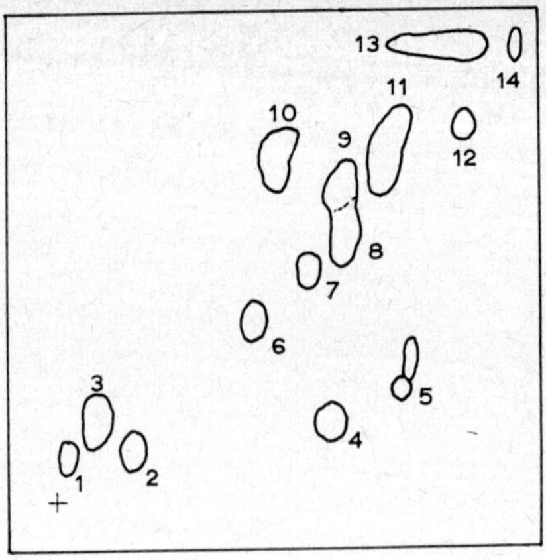

FIG. 2. Identification of the 2,4-DNP-hydrazones of the listed acids:

1 oxaloacetic
2 glyoxylic I
3 2-oxoglutaric
4 pyruvic I
5 second spots of 8, 9, 10, 11
6 glyoxylic II
7 pyruvic II
8 2-oxobutyric
9 2-oxo-4-methiolbutyric
10 p-hydroxyphenylpyruvic
11 2-oxo-isocaproate, 2-oxo-3-methylvaleric, phenylpyruvic
12 laevulinic
13 ascorbic
14 2,4-dinitrophenylhydrazine

In spot 11, three compounds coincide; since they occur in totally different metabolic diseases, this is no great drawback.

It is useful to screen the urine samples for their total amounts of keto acids before running chromatograms; the procedure is shortened compared with that of Table II and has already been published in Nyhan's textbook, (1967). The hydrazones in bicarbonate solution are estimated colorimetrically against a blank to compensate for the small amount of extracted 2,4-dinitrophenylhydrazine. The molar extinctions at 366 nm of the individual 2,4-DNPH are very similar, and the extinctions are proportional to the concentrations in the range of μmoles occurring in urine; thus the results of the screening test are not influenced by the ratio of the individual hydrazones.

The excretion of the keto acids in the urine decreases with increasing age (Fig. 3); they behave like the amino acids. Of course, there is some arbitrariness in classifying age groups, and one can see a large overlap in the mean values $\pm$ standard deviations between prematures and for

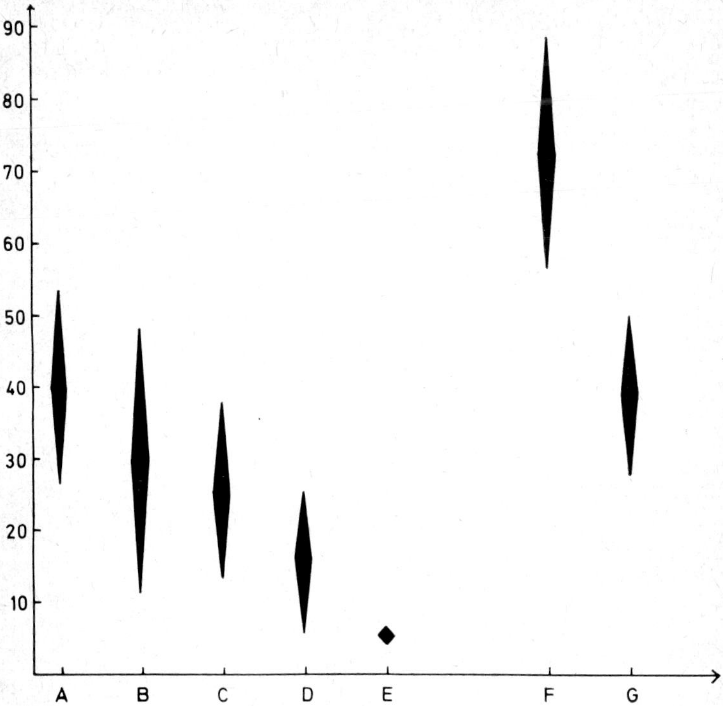

FIG. 3. Result of the screening method: Excretion of keto acids in different age groups (A-E) and diseases (F, G) in μmoles per 1 mg per cent creatinine

A: Prematures (N = 25)
B: Infants, 0–10 days (N = 43)
C: Infants, 10 days–2 months (N = 10)
D: Infants, 2 months–1 year (N = 40)
E: Children, 1–14 years (N = 25)
F: PKU and tyrosinosis (N = 11)
G: Cystinosis (N = 7)

instance 2 months old infants. An obviously significant difference exists between prematures and the group between 2 and 12 months of age. The high value of 72 ± 8 μmoles/mg per cent creatinine in phenylketonuria does not surprise. The excretion of three patients with cystinosis when measured on seven succeeding days varied between 38 and 47; 35 and 60; 22 and 28 μmoles/mg per cent creatinine, respectively, and was of the same order as that of the prematures.

Patterns of the keto acid excretion in different metabolic diseases are shown in the Figs. 4–8. At first, we look at the chromatogram of a 10 days old infant. The most intensive spot near the starting point is

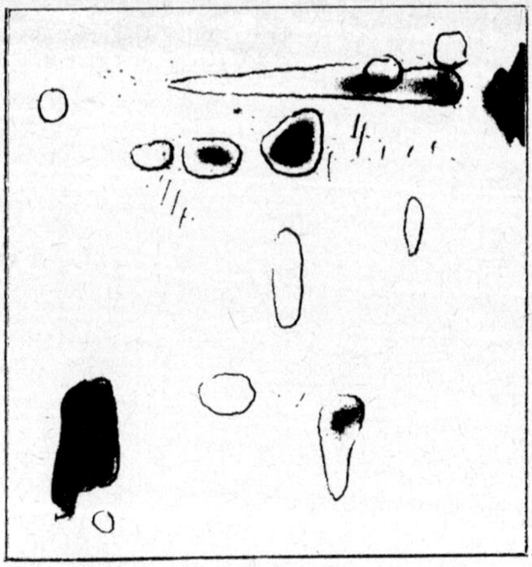

FIG. 4. α-ketoacid excretion in urine.
Infant, 10 days old, male ABO erythroblastosis, not suspicious for a metabolic disease.
TLC technique as described.

α-ketoglutaric acid. The 2,4-DNPH of pyruvic acid is to the right, in the same vertical height as α-ketoglutaric acid. The longish spot at the front represents ascorbic acid, the dark area to the right is a residue of non-extracted 2,4-dinitrophenylhydrazine. The spot below ascorbic acid is 4-hydroxyphenylpyruvic acid. In our estimation, these substances amount to about 95–98 per cent of the total keto acid present; minor spots, for instance within the ascorbic acid area and to the left of hydroxyphenyl-

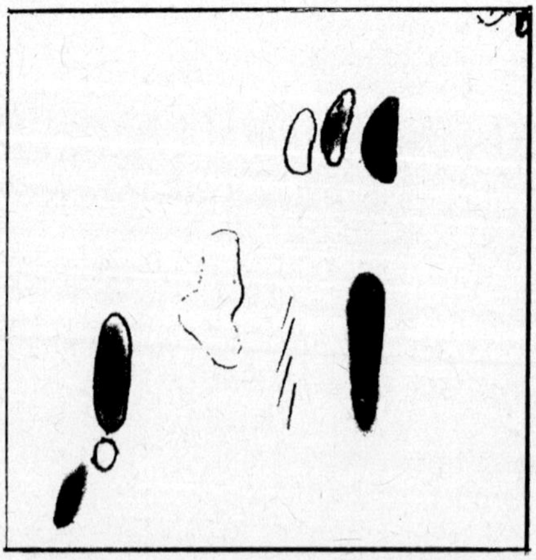

FIG. 5. α-ketoacid excretion in PKU.
Patient Th. K., male, 3 years old; TLC technique as described.

pyruvic acid were not identical with any of the keto acids tested. With increasing age, pyruvic acid may disappear totally, and the α-keto acid excretion is practically all accounted for by ketoglutaric acid excretion.

In untreated phenylketonuria the pattern (Fig. 5) is rather uniform in all patients tested. Near the starting point we recognize 2-oxoglutaric acid, to the right pyruvic acid. The four other spots form the typical pattern, the most intensive representing the two isomers of phenylpyruvic acid, the left one within the group of three is p-hydroxyphenylpyruvic acid, the middle one could not be identified precisely; possibly it is o-hydroxyphenylpyruvic acid. On a diet restricted in phenylalanine (Fig. 6) the typical pattern disappears: only faint spots close to the right-hand margin and ketoglutaric and pyruvic acids persist.

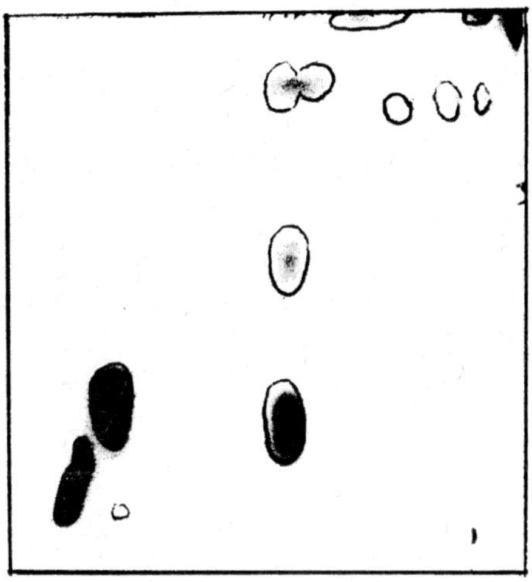

FIG. 6. α-ketoacid excretion in PKU under treatment with a diet. Patient Th. K. male, 3 years old; TLC technique as described.

In heterozygotes during a loading test, the excretion of keto acids did not rise. In one case of tyrosinosis, the total excretion of keto acids was strongly elevated with 89 μmoles/mg per cent creatinine; a substance with the chromatographic properties of p-hydroxyphenylpyruvic acid was excreted in large amounts.

The patients with cystinosis also show a rather typical α-keto acid excretion (Fig. 7). The spot close to the point of application is ketoglutaric acid. Pyruvic acid also was increased in a boy aged 4 years. In normal children, this substance disappears after the first year of life. The shape of the spot with points and tailing might suggest the presence of a second substance, but it can be proved that it is merely an overloading effect.

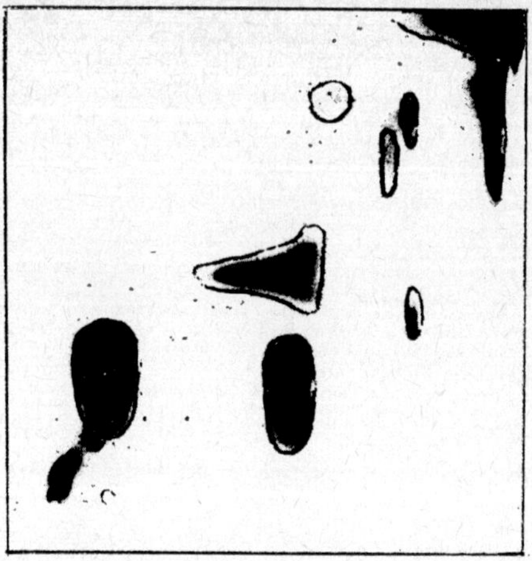

FIG. 7. α-ketoacid excretion in cystinosis. Patient Th. D., male, 4 years old; TLC technique as described.

None of the group of four spots is identical with any of the keto acids tested by us, including 2-oxo-4-methiolbutyric and 2-oxobutyric acids as metabolites of methionine. The deaminated cysteine, 2-oxo-3-sulphhydro-propionic acid, cannot be synthesised according to Master's procedure, because the sulphhydryl group is oxidised by the catalase necessary in the reaction mixture. We had hoped to find an additional parameter to check for a beneficial effect of a diet restricted in cystine and methionine; but the excretion on such a diet turned out to be just as high as when off the diet (Fig. 8).

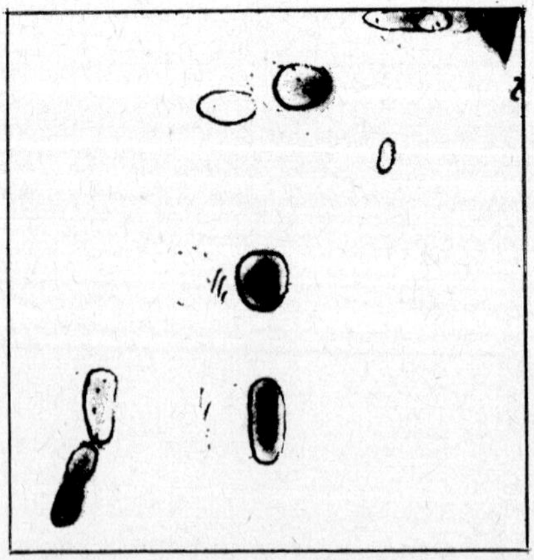

FIG. 8. α-ketoacid excretion in cystinosis under treatment with a methionine- and cystine-restricted diet. Patient Th. D., male, 4 years old; TLC technique as described.

In a case of cystinosis in an adult, the α-keto acid excretion was about normal and added one argument to the hypothesis that the metabolic condition in this variant is totally different from that in cystinosis in childhood.

In several cases of homocystinuria, we looked for the metabolites of methionine with a keto group, e.g. 2-oxo-4-sulphhydrobyturic acid, 2-oxobutyric acid, and deaminated methionine still linked to adenosine, but there were no abnormalities in the chromatogram. From this one could infer that no appreciable amount of methionine is excreted in the form of a keto acid.

In some metabolic diseases, the chromatographic pattern of the α-keto acids can apparently help to establish the diagnosis and to monitor the effect of dietary treatment.

REFERENCES

BAYZER, H. (1971) *J. Chromatogr.*, **57**, 275.

BERLET, H. H. (1968) *Anal. Biochem.*, **22**, 525.

CAVALLINI, D., FRONTALI, N. & TOSCHI, G. (1949) *Nature*, **164**, 792.

COTTE, J., COLLOMBEL, C., CUIVRE, M. & PADIS, L. (1967) *Rev. Fr. Etudes clin. biol.*, **12**, 496.

COWARD, R. F., SMITH, P. & SEAKINS, J. W. T. (1969) *J. clin. Path.*, **22**, 422.

COWARD, R. F. & SMITH, P. (1968) *J. Chromatogr.*, **33**, 508.

DANCIS, J., HUTZLER, J. & LEVITZ, M. (1963) *Biochem. Biophys. Acta.*, **78**, 85.

KÄSER, H., KÄSER, R. & LESTRADET, H. (1960) *Metabolism*, **9**, 926.

LUTZ, P., & V. REUTERN, G. M. (1969) *Z. klin. Chem. u. klin. Biochem.*, **7**, 586.

MENKES, J. H. (1960) *Am. J. Dis. child.*, **99**, 500.

NYHAN, W. L. (ed.) *Amino Acid Metabolism and Genetic Variation*. New York, Toronto, London, Sydney: The Blakiston Division, McGraw-Hill Book Company, p. 461: TOCCI, P. M. (1967).

RONKAINEN, P. (1967) *J. Chromatogr.*, **28**, 440.

RONKAINEN, P. (1967) *J. Chromatogr.*, **28**, 259.

SAINI, A. S. (1967) *J. Chromatogr.*, **26**, 539.

SMITH, P. (1967) *J. Chromatogr.*, **30**, 273.

STAN, H.-J. & SCHORMÜLLER, J. (1969) *J. Chromatogr.*, **43**, 103.

THE USE OF DEUTERATED PHENYLALANINE FOR THE ELUCIDATION OF THE PHENYLALANINE-TYROSINE METABOLISM

by

H.-CH. CURTIUS, J. A. VÖLLMIN AND K. BAERLOCHER

Introduction

THE use of radioactive isotopes as metabolic tracers in man is not without risk and only in certain cases can it be justified. The application of radioactive, stable isotopes, e.g. ^{15}N, ^{13}C or deuterium was rarely used until now because the measurement of such isotopes presented some analytical problems (Schoenheimer & Rittenberg, 1935).

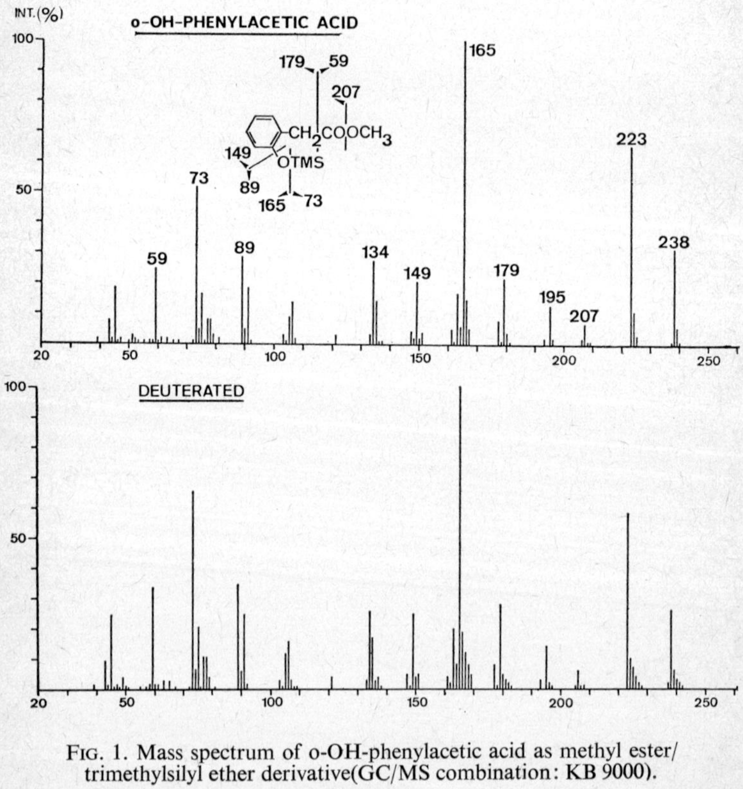

FIG. 1. Mass spectrum of o-OH-phenylacetic acid as methyl ester/trimethylsilyl ether derivative(GC/MS combination: KB 9000).

The most suitable instrument for the detection of stable isotopes is the mass spectrometer. The application of mass spectrometric isotope measurements is demonstrated with the example of o-OH-phenylacetic acid, an important excretion product in phenylketonuria. Fig. 1 shows the mass spectrum of o-OH-phenylacetic acid as methyl ester/trimethylsilyl ether derivative.

The formation of derivatives is necessary because the mass spectrum is recorded in combination with a gas chromatograph. After separation, the quantitation of isotope abundance is done on the molecular signal if its amount is high enough. By replacement with deuterium, peaks with higher masses are observed as can be seen in Fig. 2.

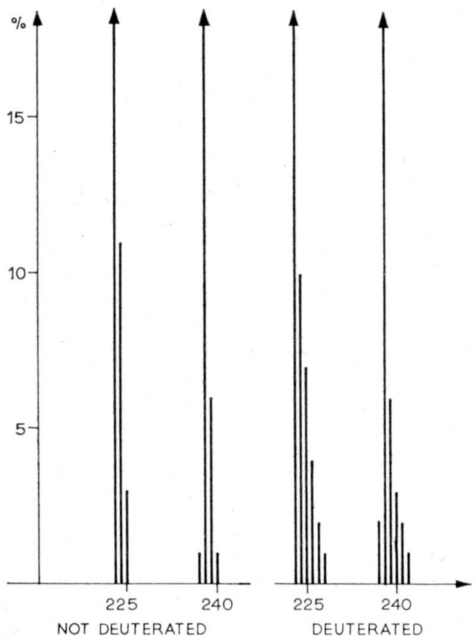

FIG. 2. Comparison of higher masses of o-OH-phenylacetic acid (see Fig. 1).

The separation and purification of the different compounds is very troublesome and usually results in an inadequate yield. However, since the introduction of the combined gas chromatograph/mass spectrometer a few years ago, this problem has been simplified (Holmes *et al.*, 1957; Ryhage, 1964). Complicated biological mixtures can thus be separated and analysed in a combination of gas chromatograph/mass spectrometer: The effluent of the gas chromatograph is directly fed into the mass spectrometer for isotope measurements (Pinkus *et al.*, 1971).

Results

Fig. 3 shows a gas chromatographic separation of a test mixture of

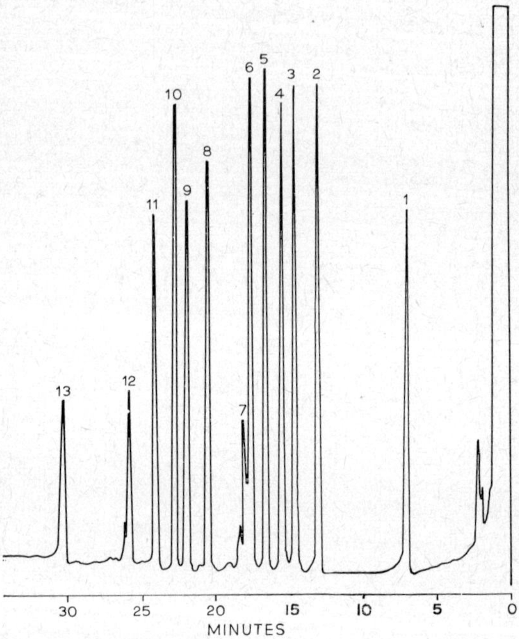

FIG. 3. GLC separation of a test mixture of aromatic acids as methyl esters/trimethylsilyl derivatives;
gas chromatograph: Aerograph model 1520;
column conditions: XE 60 3 per cent on Chromosorb G 80-10 mesh;
glass column 2 m, i.d. 2·7 mm
t_c: 110°C, 5 min isotherm; heating rate: 4°C/min
to 200°C; t_i: 230°C; t_d: 220°C; N_2: 45 ml/min.

1 Phenylacetic acid
2 Mandelic acid
3 Phenyllactic acid
4 o-OH-Phenylacetic acid
5 m-OH-Phenylacetic acid
6 p-OH-Phenylacetic acid
7 Phenylpyruvic acid
8 m-OH-Phenylhydracrylic acid
9 Homovanillic acid
10 p-OH-Phenyllactic acid
11 Vanillylmandelic acid
12 p-OH-Phenylpyruvic acid
13 Hippuric acid

these metabolites as methyl esters/trimethylsilyl ethers by the method of Völlmin *et al.*, 1971.

The gas chromatographic profile of the urinary aromatic acids in a healthy child is given in Fig. 4.

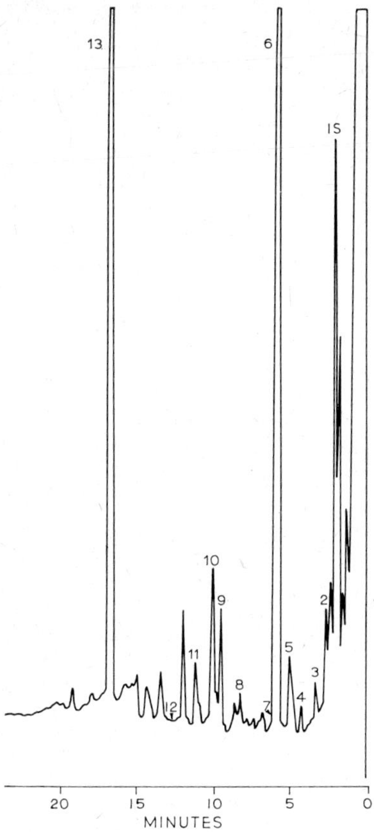

FIG. 4. GLC separation of urinary aromatic acids of a normal child aged 9 months (derivatives and GLC conditions see Fig. 3).

2 Mandelic acid
3 Phenyllactic acid
4 o-OH-Phenylacetic acid
5 m-OH-Phenylacetic acid
6 p-OH-Phenylacetic acid
7 Phenylpyruvic acid
8 m-OH-Phenylhydracrylic acid
9 Homovanillic acid
10 p-OH-Phenyllactic acid
11 Vanillylmandelic acid
12 p-OH-Phenylpyruvic acid
13 Hippuric acid

The main metabolites are p-OH-phenylacetic acid, homovanillic acid, p-OH-phenyllactic acid, and hippuric acid.

The urinary profile of a patient with phenylketonuria (PKU) is presented in Fig. 5.

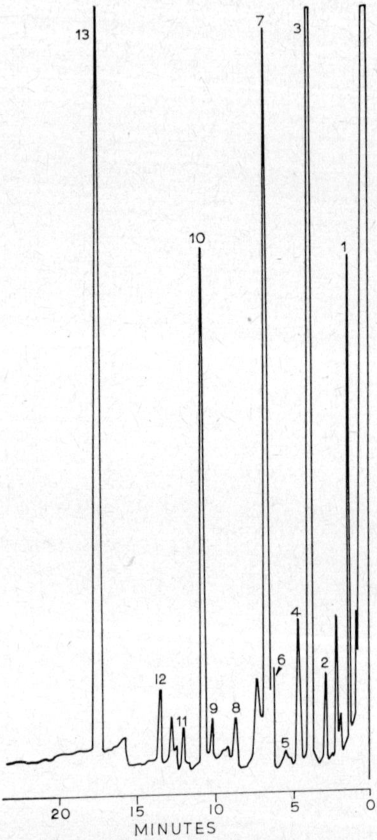

FIG. 5. GLC separation of urinary aromatic acids of a patient with PKU aged 14 days; (urine collected just prior to beginning of diet) (derivatives and GLC conditions see Fig. 3).

1 Phenylacetic acid
2 Mandelic acid
3 Phenyllactic acid
4 o-OH-Phenylacetic acid
5 m-OH-Phenylacetic acid
6 p-OH-Phenylacetic acid
7 Phenylpyruvic acid
8 m-OH-Phenylhydracrylic acid
9 Homovanillic acid
10 p-OH-Phenyllactic acid
11 Vanillylmandelic acid
12 p-OH-Phenylpyruvic acid
13 Hippuric acid

Metabolites present in high concentrations are: phenylacetic acid, phenyllactic acid, o-OH-phenylacetic acid, phenylpyruvic acid, but the p-hydroxylated compounds (p-OH-phenyllactic acid, p-OH-phenylpyruvic acid) and finally hippuric acid are also increased.

Three subjects were studied, a normal child (age 3 years), a patient with PKU (age: 12 5/12 years; plasma phenylalanine concentration: 25 mg/100 ml), and a patient with hyperphenylalaninaemia (age: 1 4/12 years; plasma phenylalanine concentration: 7 mg/100 ml). These three subjects were orally loaded with 200 mg/kg body weight of 27 per cent deuterated DL-phenylalanine.*

We then studied two different variables: concentration changes of phenylalanine and tyrosine and their metabolites, and, secondly, the deuterium distribution pattern among the metabolic pathways.

Loading with Deuterated Phenylalanine

Concentration of metabolites and amino acids

Fig. 6 demonstrates the increase of phenylalanine in plasma and urine during the loading test.

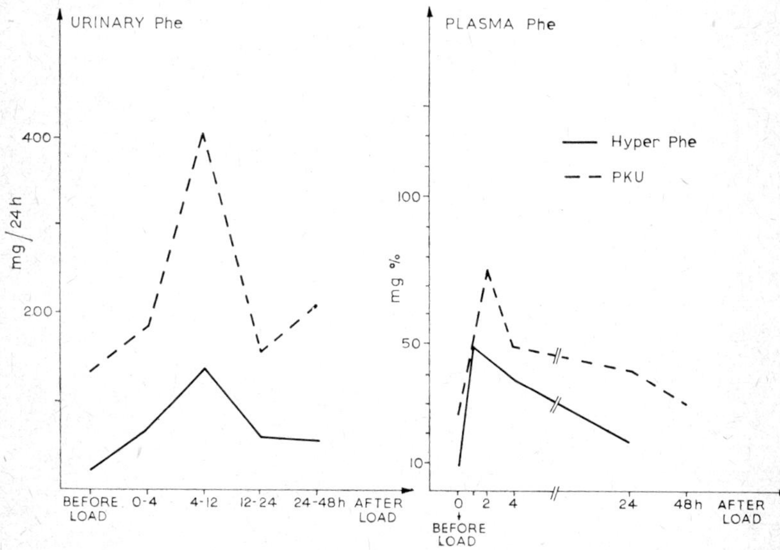

FIG. 6. Urinary and plasma phenylalanine concentration during loading with 200 mg/kg DL-phenylalanine.

In the patient with PKU as well as in the patient with hyperphenylalaninaemia, tyrosine in urine was found in very small quantities.

* Purchased from ISOCOMMERZ, Leipzig.

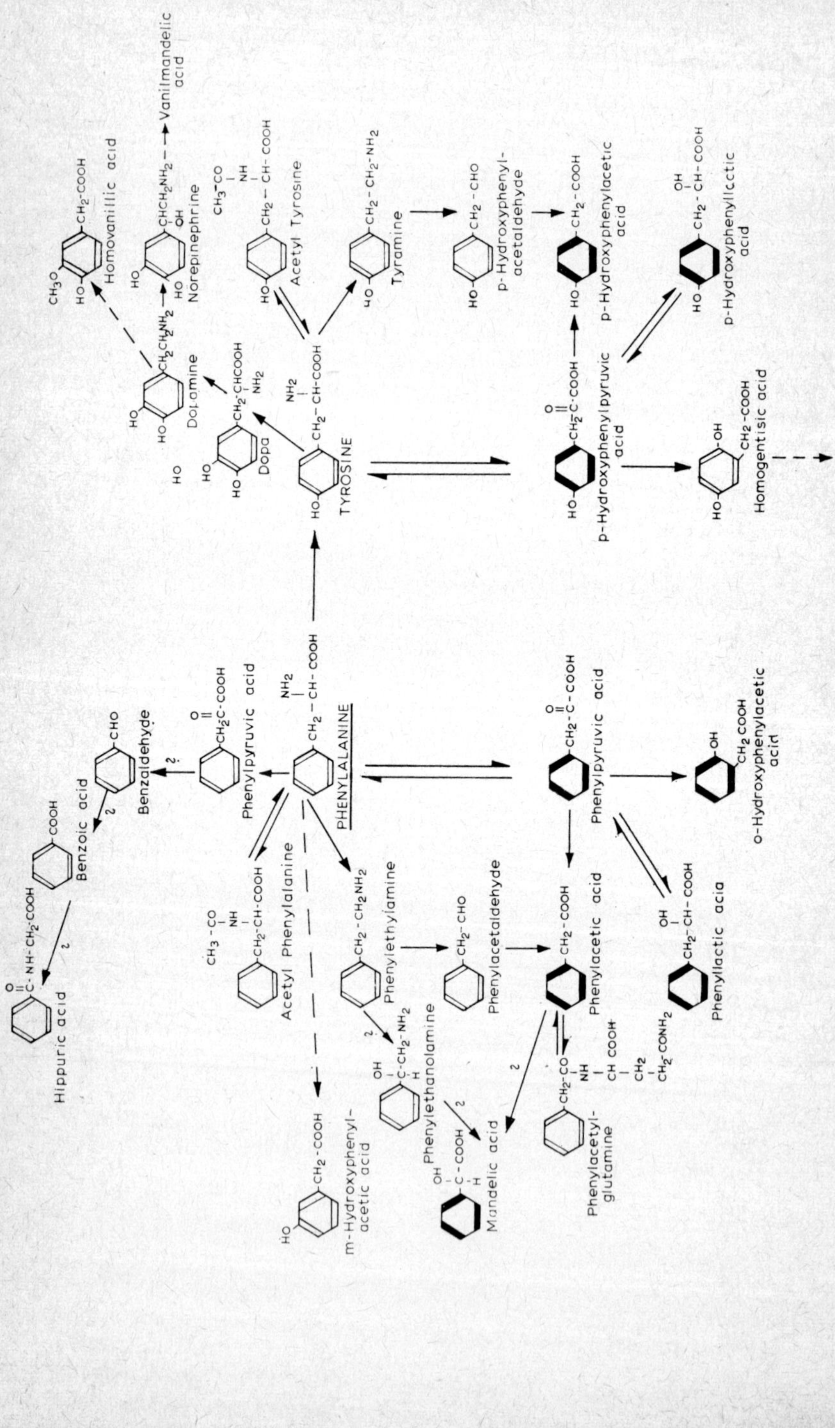

FIG. 7. Normal subject: loading with phenylalanine (increased metabolites are marked).

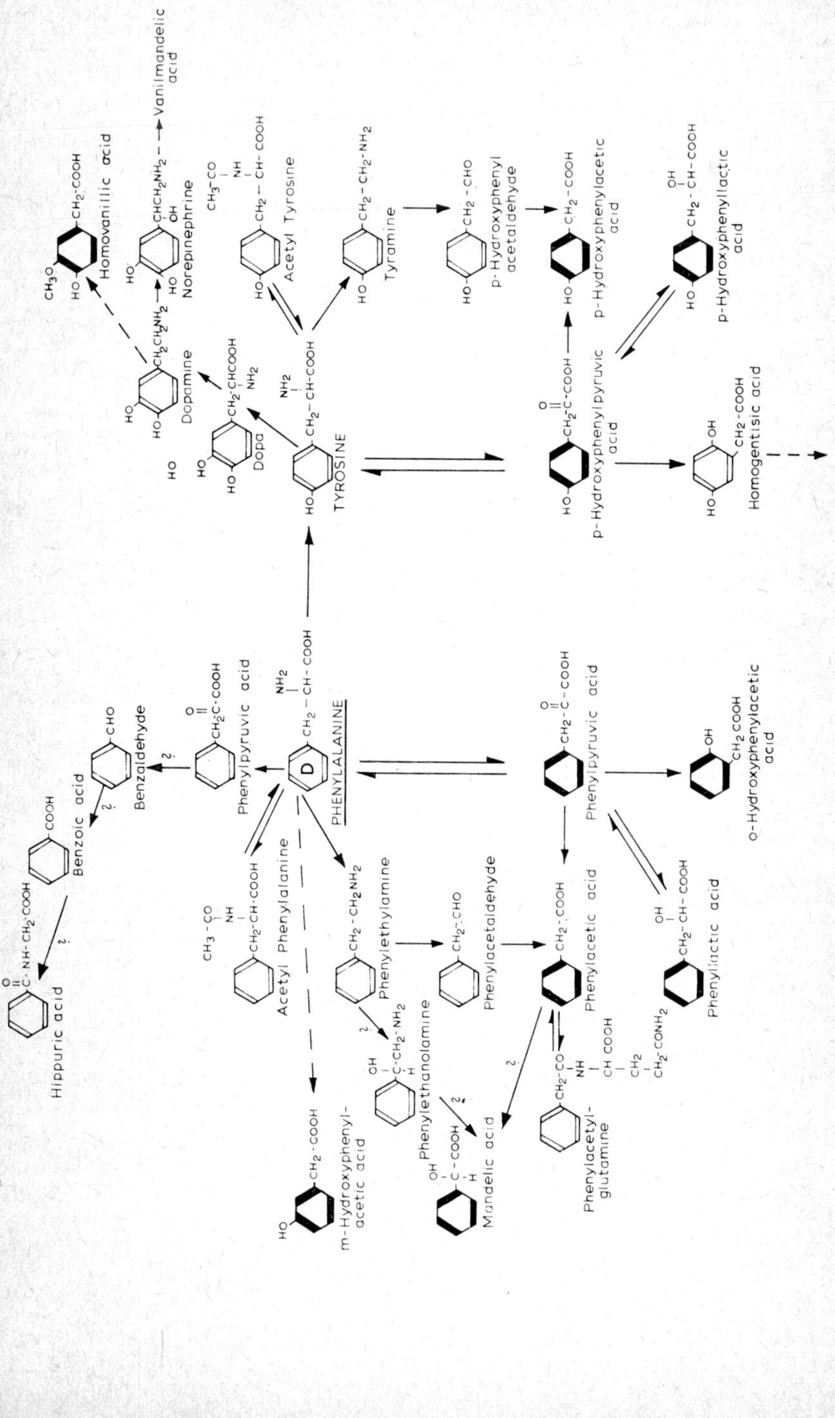

FIG. 8. Normal subject: loading with deuterated phenylalanine (deuterium labelled compounds are marked).

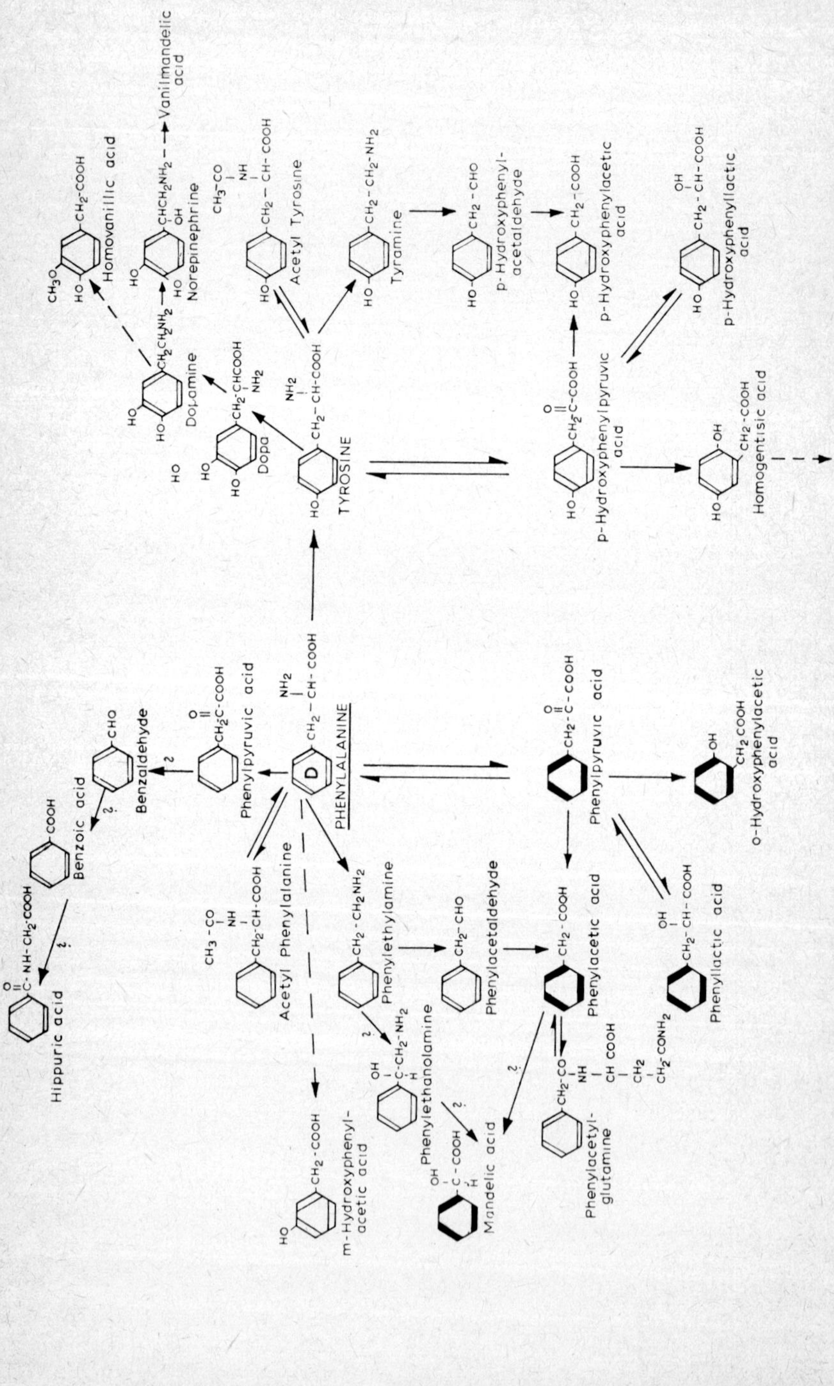

FIG. 9. Phenylketonuria: loading with deuterated phenylalanine (deuterium labelled compounds are marked).

Fig. 7 shows the urinary aromatic acids from the phenylalanine tyrosine metabolism of a healthy child.

The following metabolites are increased phenylpyruvic acid, phenyllactic acid, phenylacetic acid, o-OH-phenylacetic acid, mandelic acid (first described by Blau, 1970), p-OH-phenylpyruvic acid, p-OH-phenyllactic acid, and p-OH-phenylacetic acid.

A similar pattern but a higher increase of these metabolites was found in the case of PKU after a phenylalanine load. The unexpectedly high excretion of p-OH-phenyllactic acid and p-OH-phenylpyruvic acid has already been reported by other investigators (Knox, 1966).

Labelling patterns

Figs. 8 and 9 present our results after a load with deuterated phenylalanine. The former shows the excretion products of a healthy child. It should be emphasised that m-OH-phenylacetic acid, mandelic acid and homovanillic acid are also considerably deuterated. In contrast, however, the situation in the case of PKU is different (Fig. 9).

No deuterium incorporation could be detected here in the metabolites of tyrosine; p-OH-phenylpyruvic acid, p-OH-phenyllactic acid, p-OH-phenylacetic acid and homovanillic acid could not be found deuterated. It is of special interest, that m-OH-phenylacetic acid was not deuterated. Mandelic acid on the other hand was still deuterated to about the same extent as in the healthy child.

These results raise some interesting questions with respect to the importance of the various pathways involved (see discussion).

In the patient with hyperphenylalaninaemia, the same deuteration pattern was observed as in the PKU patient.

Concentration and deuteration pattern of o-OH-phenylacetic acid, phenyllactic acid, and p-OH-phenyllactic acid in different periods of urine collection after load

In the three subjects the concentration and deuterium content of some metabolites during the loading test is presented in Figs. 10 and 11.

During loading with deuterated phenylalanine, o-OH-phenylacetic acid was excreted in increased amounts and with the same deuteration profile in the three subjects.

A very similar pattern was found for phenyllactic acid. It is remarkable, that these metabolites showed the same increase in hyperphenylalaninaemia as in PKU. The basal value, however, was considerably lower in the hyperphenylalaninaemic patient.

Finally, Fig. 11 shows the rather remarkable pattern found for p-OH-phenyllactic acid. Its concentration increased in all three subjects just as with the immediate metabolites of phenylalanine shown above, but deuteration is found only in the healthy child.

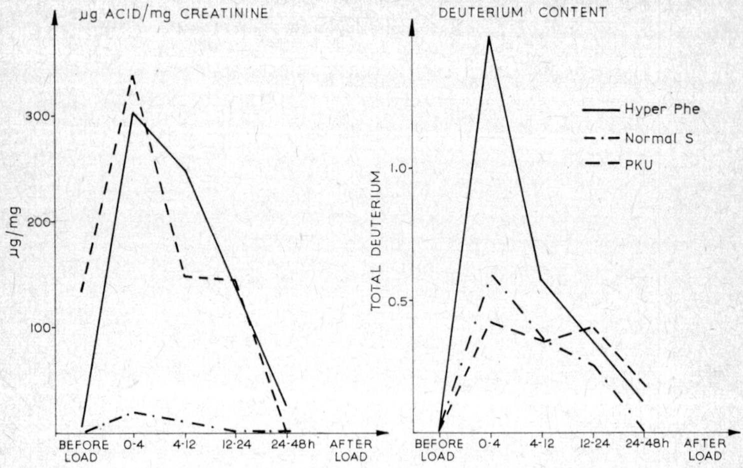

FIG. 10. Urinary excretion of o-OH-phenylactic acid after deuterated phenylalanine load (200 mg/kg).

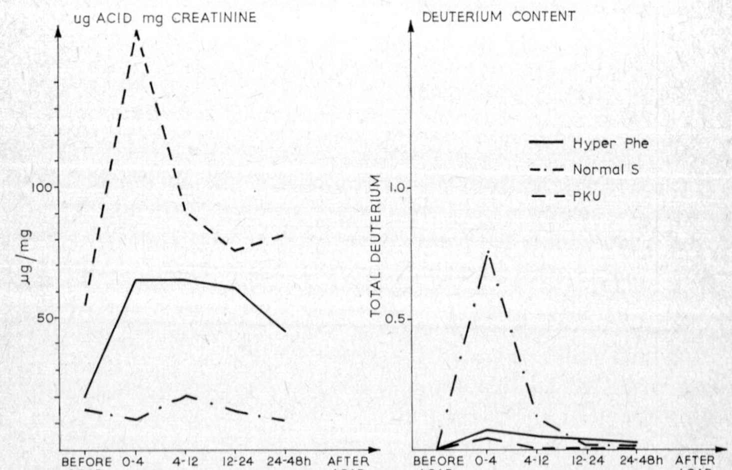

FIG. 11. Urinary excretion of p-OH-phenylactic acid after deuterated phenylalanine load (200 mg/kg).

Discussion and Conclusions

These investigations up to now show some interesting features:

1. Blau (1970) was the first to report the presence of mandelic acid in PKU. We found that mandelic acid is also present in metabolically healthy subjects after a phenylalanine load. The marked labelling of mandelic acid after loading with deuterated phenylalanine proves the hypothesis that it is definitely a product of phenylalanine metabolism.
2. The fact that we were unable to detect any deuteration of hippuric acid suggests that hippuric acid is synthesised mainly from alimentary benzoic acid and not through the phenylalanine/phenylpyruvic acid pathway.
3. It is well known that in PKU p-hydroxylated metabolites, e.g. p-OH-phenyllactic acid and p-OH-phenylpyruvic acid are elevated (Knox 1966). In PKU, no deuterium was found in p-hydroxylated compounds. This lack of deuteration shows rather unambiguously that the enzyme block between phenylalanine and tyrosine cannot be circumvented by other metabolic connections and would therefore substantiate the hypothesis that a secondary inhibition due to the metabolites of phenylalanine does take place.
4. In the healthy child, homovanillic acid, the main metabolite of dopamine was deuterated whereas in PKU this compound showed no deuterium incorporation. In addition, the concentration of homovanillic acid was markedly decreased in patients with PKU (Völlmin *et al.*, 1971). In this connection, the question arises once more, whether the lack of tyrosine metabolites, e.g. of the biologically active amines and homovanillic acid may contribute to the impairment of brain function.
5. In the healthy subject, m-OH-phenylacetic acid was markedly deuterated, but practically not in patients with PKU. It seems that in PKU, m-hydroxylation of phenylacetic acid is blocked. We would like to point to the fact that m-hydroxylation of tyrosine is catalysed by tyrosine-3-hydroxylase, and that several inhibitors of this enzyme are known, one of which is phenylalanine (Nagatsu *et al.*, 1964).
6. A patient with hyperphenylalaninaemia, whose plasma phenylalanine was 7·0 mg/100 ml before load, showed the same deuteration pattern as the patient with PKU with a plasma phenylalanine of 25 mg/100 ml. In the former, the concentration of the metabolites and of phenylalanine itself was lower before and during the loading test. The lack of deuteration of tyrosine metabolites makes it obvious that in our patient with hyperphenylalaninaemia, no phenylalanine or nearly none is metabolized to tyrosine. The lower phenylalanine concentration and the lower concentration of its metabolites might suggest that another metabolic pathway for phenylalanine degradation exists in patients with hyperphenylalaninaemia.

In conclusion, the present investigation shows that the stable isotope technique may be a powerful instrument for the study of metabolic pathways in man.

REFERENCES

BLAU, K. (1970) *Clin. chim. Acta*, **27**, 5.
HOLMES, J. C., & MORELL F. A. (1957) *Appl. Spectrosc.*, **11**, 86.
KNOX, W. E. (1966) *In Metabolic Basis of Inherited Disease*, J. B. Stanbury, J. B. Wyngaarden & D. S. Fredrickson, (eds.). McGraw-Hill, p. 258.
NAGATSU, T., LEVITT, M. & UDENFRIED, S. (1964) *J. biol. Chem.*, **239**, 2910.
PINKUS, J. L., CHARLES, D. & CHATTORAJ, S. C. (1971) *J. biol. Chem.*, **246**, 633.
RYHAGE, R. (1964) *Analyt. Chem.*, **36**, 959.
SCHOENHEIMER, R. & RITTENBERG, D. (1935) *J. biol. Chem.*, **111**, 163.
VÖLLMIN, J. A. BOSSHARD, H. R., MÜLLER, M., RAMPINI, S. & CURTIUS, H.-CH. (1971) *Z. klin. Chem. u. klin. Biochem.*, **9**, 402.

DISCUSSION
(of Papers by Dr Lutz and Dr Curtius)

La Du (*New York*). DL-phenylalanine may show a different pattern of labelled metabolite from that of L-phenylalanine. It would be important to repeat the deuterium experiments with the latter.

Curtius (*Zurich*). Experiments with L-phenylalanine now are in progress. For the work reported here, the L-form was not yet at our disposal.

Seakins (*London*). D-phenylalanine is metabolised and handled differently from L-phenylalanine in the homozygous normal subject (J. W. T. Seakins, 1971, *Clin. Chim. Acta*). Is not a loading dose of deuterated DL-phenylalanine going to result in a complex pattern? Did you examine deuteration patterns in phenylacetylglutamine? Is not m-hydroxylation a characteristic of gut-flora metabolism?

Curtius. As already mentioned we shall also start loading tests with deuterated L-phenylalanine. Up to now we have not yet investigated phenylacetylglutamine. m-Hydroxylation will mainly be effected by endogenous enzyme action, either directly from phenylalanine or indirectly via tyrosine, dopamine, the 4-OH group being removed by a dehydroxylating enzyme.

Bickel (*Heidelberg*). Dr Curtius, am I right in concluding that with your sensitive and specific methods you found no qualitative differences between classical phenylketonuria and so-called hyperphenylalaninaemia in phenolic acid excretion?

Curtius. Yes, in our patients we could only find the quantitative difference in the concentration of the metabolites, but we hope that loading tests with deuterated L-tyrosine will answer this question.

INVESTIGATION OF TRYPTOPHAN METABOLISM IN PATIENTS WITH UNTREATED PHENYLKETONURIA

by

W. Kochen, D. Byrd and R. Bühner

Tryptophan metabolism was analysed in ten patients who had been recognised to be phenylketonurics in serial Guthrie tests carried out in the Johannes-Anstalten at Mosbach, Federal Republic of Germany. Three patients had been treated clinically at the University Children's Hospital in Heidelberg. But the diet-therapy had proved unsuccessful and had been discontinued. The case histories of the seven other patients are incomplete. Their anamneses, however, are typical for phenylketonurics.

The ten patients were divided on the basis of their phenylalanine values into two groups, those with values below 20 mg per cent and those with values exceeding this level.

For analytical reasons we subdivided the metabolites of tryptophan into three groups:

(I) the oxidative degradation products of the kynurenine pathway leading to 3-hydroxyanthranilic acid;
(II) those from the metabolism of 3-hydroxyanthranilic acid to nicotinamide and its metabolites especially N_1-methyl-2-pyridone-5-carboxamide;
(III) the indole metabolites.

I. The Kynurenine Pathway

For the exact identification and quantitative determination of the oxidative degradation products we used column, thin layer, and gas chromatography, and mass spectrometry. This combination enables us to observe the appearance of new and unknown metabolites. This type of work up also makes it possible to see general and specific differences between urine obtained before and after loading with tryptophan.

The results of this analysis led us to divide the patients into two groups, A and B. Group A contains all of the patients with high values in the Guthrie-test and one with a lower value. In group B there are only those patients with lower Guthrie-test values. In Table I are shown the mean values for the excreted metabolites obtained in both groups. Contrary to control urines none of the patients excrete 3-hydroxyanthranilic acid in

Table I. *Mean urinary excretion (mg/24 hours) of tryptophan metabolites of the kynurenine pathway in patients with untreated phenylketonuria. 0·1 g L-tryptophan/kg body weight*
b = basal urine, l = first 24 hrs. after loading, Ky = kynurenine, KyA = kynurenic acid, 3-OH-Ky = 3-hydroxykynurenine, XA = xanthurenic acid, 3-OH-AA = 3-hydroxyanthranilic acid, AA = anthranilic acid, Try = tryptophan

Metabolite	Group A (n = 7) b	l	Group B (n = 3) b	l	Controls (n = 12) b	l
Ky	1·09 (0–3·27)	5·45 (0.51–17.78	1·33 (1·00–1·66)	99·14 (56·68–149·05)	1·5±0·7	15·0±6·0
KyA	2·33 (0–6·03)	7·80 (3·09–17·52)	5·29 (3·25–6·94)	79·39 (41·93–109·25)	1·78±1·4	12·9±7·3
3-OH-Ky	0·61 (0–3·36)	2·09 (0–5·12)	3·73 (0–7·20)	92·74 (58·80–134·01)	1·35±0·3	6·8±4·5
XA	0·53 (0–1·13)	4·60 (0·65–15·05)	2·03 (1·35–2·85)	34·12 (27·16–46·15)	0·95±0·4	7·4±2·0
3-OH-AA	0	0	0	7·00 (2·33–11·90)	0·6±0·3	4·5±1·5
AA	0	0	0	0	0	0–1 mg
% of Try dose		0·65 (0·23–1·03)		4·84 (4·09–5·71)		2·0±0·6

the pre-load urine. After tryptophan loading this metabolite is excreted only in group B. These values exceed that of controls.

It is seen that under tryptophan loading group B shows, in sharp contrast to group A, a large increase in excretion of metabolites which far exceeds that of the controls. The ratios of the mean after-load values to the mean basal values make the difference between the two groups even more obvious (see Table II). In group B the excretion of the metabolites

Table II. *Ratio of mean urinary values before and after tryptophan loading:*
Ky=kynurenine, KyA=kynurenic acid, 3-OH-Ky = 3-hydroxykynurenine, XA = xanthurenic acid

Metabolite	*Group A*	*Group B*	*Controls*
Ky	5·0	75·0	10·0
KyA	3·3	15·0	7·2
3-OH-Ky	3·4	24·9	5·0
XA	8·7	16·8	7·8

kynurenine, kynurenic acid, 3-hydroxykynurenine and xanthurenic acid is respectively 15, 5, 7 and 2 times as great as in group A.

The patients of group B are further characterised by excretion, especially after tryptophan loading, of several chemically related, highly fluorescent compounds. One of these, when isolated, proved to be very labile in the presence of strong acids or when heated. Under these conditions it was broken down into o-aminoacetophenone and an unidentified component. The examination of the original compound (X_1 or X_2 in Fig. 1) by the combination of gas chromatography and mass spectrometry revealed only the cleavage product o-amineacetophenone. Fig. 1 presents a proposal for the biogenesis. It should be noted that this group of chemically related compounds are not found in the urines of group A.

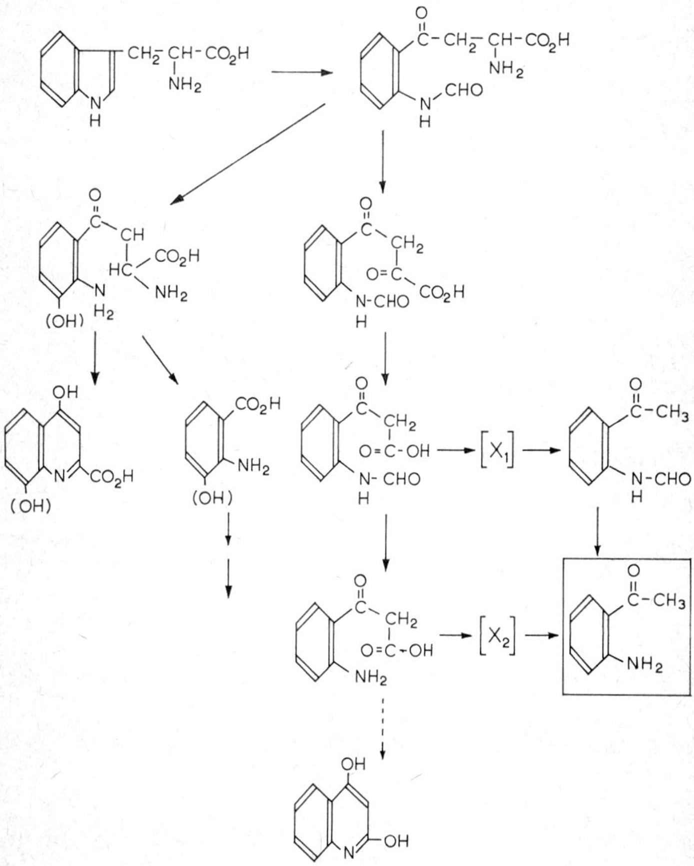

FIG. 1. Proposed pathway for the biogenesis of o-aminoacetophenone.

Special attention should be paid to the excretion of two quinoline derivatives. So far the 8-hydroxy derivative of quinaldic acid could not be found in normal urine. In four of the phenylketonurics considerable amounts of both quinaldic acid and 8-hydroxyquinaldic acid could be detected. The excretion of quinaldic acid in the basal urine ranges from 4 to 10 mg/24 hours and after loading from 14 to 170 mg. The range for 8-hydroxyquinaldic acid in basal urine is from 2 to 8 mg/24 hours. It is not greatly increased by tryptophan loading. The discovery of these compounds is of interest as they indicate the existence of an "unphysiological" dehydroxylation of xanthurenic and kynurenic acid. Until now 8-hydroxyquinaldic acid has been found in urine only in the case of a child suffering from vitamin B_6-dependent seizures. This metabolite could be detected in urine after the B_6 therapy had been discontinued. It is suspected that a connection exists between the seizures and the appearance of 8-hydroxyquinaldic acid in the urine (Kochen, 1971).

II. Metabolites of 3-Hydroxyanthranilic Acid

For this second group of metabolites it was necessary to develop a new method for individual separation and identification. This will be published in detail shortly. The analytical difficulties with this group of metabolites stem mainly from the fact that apart from König's reagent for nicotinic acid there is no specific staining reagent for the other members of the group. The method developed includes the quantitative determination of the following metabolites: quinolinic acid, nicotinic acid, picolinic acid, nicotinamide, N_1-methylnicotinamide, nicotinuric acid, nicotinamide-N-oxide, nicotinic acid -N-oxide, N_1-methyl-2-pyridone-5-carboxylic acid and its amide, N_1-methyl-4-pyridone-5-carboxamide and 2-hydroxypyridine-5-carboxylic acid.

The results obtained from the analysis of these metabolites in four of the patients are shown in Table III. The lack of quinolinic acid is especially noteworthy. Picolinic acid, 2-hydroxypyridine-5-carboxylic acid, nicotinic acid-N-Oxide and N_1-methyl-2-pyridone-5-carboxylic acid were

Table III. *Urinary excretion of tryptophan metabolites resulting from the metabolism of 3-hydroxyanthranilic acid in subjects with untreated phenylketonuria (mg/24 hours).* Quin. A = quinolinic acid, N_1MNAA = N_1-methylnicotinamide, 2PyAAM, = N_1 methyl-2-pyridone-5-carboxamide, NicA = nicotinic acid, NicAAm = nicotinamide, NicA-Gly = nicotinuric acid, NicAAm-NO = nicotinamide-N-Oxide, 4 PyAAm = N_1-methyl-4-pyridone-5-carboxamide.
$+^1$ = identification not fully established.

	Group A				*Group B*			
	pat.7		pat.8		pat.9		pat.10	
Metabolite	b	l	b	l	b	l	b	l
Quin.A	0	0	0	0	0	0	0	0
N_1MNAA	4·5	7·9	7·8	10·3	4·2	10·4	2·1	3·5
2PyAAM	6·8	9·2	16·0	28·0	7·2	11·3	8·2	17·4
NicA	0	0	0	0	3·6	0	0	0
NicAAm	0	+	0	0	3·4	0·9	20·7	11·6
NicA-Gly	0	0	0	0	0	4·9	0	0
NicAAm-NO	$+^1$	$+^1$	0	0	0	0	0	0
4PYAAm	$+^1$	$+^1$	—	—	$+^1$	$+^1$	—	—

also not detected. The basal and loading results for N_1-methylnicotinamide and N_1-methyl-2-pyridone-5-carboxamide lie within the normal range. This means that this pathway of tryptophan and of 3-hydroxyanthranilic acid is unhindered in these patients.

III. Urinary Indole Compounds

The tryptophan metabolites with indole structure were extracted from urine and analysed in thin-layer and gas chromatography and mass spectrometry. A total of thirty-three indole compounds were detected in amounts exceeding 0·1 mg/24 hours. The structures of a number of these are still under investigation.

A new urinary indole whose identity has just been established is indole-3-carbaldehyde. Its structure was determined on the basis of the uv, ir and mass spectra. The mass spectrum of the isolated indole-3-aldehyde is shown in Fig. 2. The molecular peak M^+ is at 145 mass units. The $M^+ - 1$ peak, at 144 mass units, has approximately the same intensity as the molecular peak; this is characteristic of aromatic aldehydes. The loss of the carbonyl function is indicated by the peak at 116 mass units.

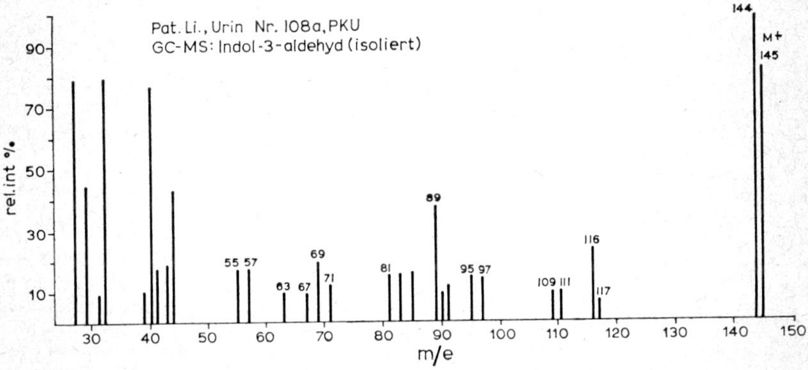

FIG. 2. Mass spectrum of indole-3-carbaldehyde.

Those indole compounds whose chemical structure could be determined were assayed. The quantitative and the qualitative results of the analysis of the indoles led again to a division of the patients into two groups A and B which correspond to the groups A and B discussed in connection with the analysis of the products of the kynurenine pathway. Table IV presents the results from two subjects who are typical for their respective groups. The A group is characterised by the comparatively poor ability to produce neutral indoles and by the absence of tryptamine. Patients in this group also did not excrete N-acetyltryptophan (with one exception where

Table IV. *Urinary excretion of indolic metabolites of tryptophan in two untreated PKU patients typical of their respective groups A and B. Identified compounds in mg/24 hours IAAm = indoleacetamide; I-3-Ald = indole-3-aldehyde, N-Ac-Tryam = N-acetyltryptamine; N-Ac-Try = N-acetyltryptophan; ILA = indolelactic acid, IAA = indoleacetic acid; I-3-CA = indolecarboxylic acid; 5-OH-IAA = 5-hydroxyindoleacetic acid.*

	Group B		*Group A*	
	b	l	b	l
Neutral indoles				
IAAm	trace	1·7	0	0
I-3-Ald	trace	1·5	0	0
N-Ac-Tryam	trace	2·0	0	0
10211 (unknown)	+	++	0	+
1088 ,,	0	++	0	0
1028 ,,	+	+	0	0
1029 ,,	0	++	0	0
10210 ,,	+	+	0	0
Basic indoles				
Tryam	trace	0·2	0	0
Serotonin	0	0	0	0
Acidic indoles				
N-Ac-Try	21·5	190·0	0	0
ILA	22·2	61·0	12·3	12·3
IAA	21·6	54·8	3·1	1·3
I-3-CA	3·4	3·0	2·8	3·0
5-OH-IAA	3·2	3·8	0	0
1023 (unknown)	trace	++	0	0
1026 ,,	0	++	0	0
10812 ,,	++	++	0	0
Amphoteric indoles				
Try	4·6	52·7	10·5	4·3

modest amounts were found). Tryptophan loading causes only insignificant increases in excretion. It can be seen that there is less excretion of some metabolites under tryptophan loading than under basal conditions.

Group B on the other hand shows a rich excretion pattern especially of neutral compounds. Most of the substances are increased significantly by a tryptophan load. The metabolic activity here is comparable to that observed in the study of the oxidative degradation in group B. The level of urinary tryptophan is raised significantly by a tryptophan load in group B. Noteworthy, however, is the excretion of the serotonin metabolite 5-hydroxyindoleacetic acid which is found in small amounts in the basal urine. Tryptophan loading has no effect on the excretion of this metabolite.

When the results obtained from the analysis of each of the three groups of tryptophan metabolites are compared, it appears that the analysis of the urinary indoles offers the best hope of differentiating between the two groups of PKU patients. Further investigation will determine how general this method of classification is.

DISCUSSION
(of the Paper by Dr Byrd)

Berry (*Cincinnati*). Were tryptophan loading tests repeated after administration of vitamin B_6?

Byrd (*Heidelberg*). Your question is supposedly based on the opinion that vitamin B_6 deficiency is manifested by abnormal xanthurenic acid formation under tryptophan loading.

We have not done a tryptophan loading experiment with simultaneous vitamin B_6 supplementation. Our primary interest was to obtain an overall picture of tryptophan metabolism in untreated phenylketonuria under normal dietary conditions. The possibility of vitamin B_6 influence did not occur to us at the very beginning of the experiments. However, at that time the determination of serum vitamin B_6 in three of the patients revealed normal levels of pyridoxal-5-phosphate. On the other hand we are not convinced of the validity of the xanthurenic acid test for vitamin B_6 deficiency. To our knowledge no exact correlation between xanthurenic acid formation and serum pyridoxal-5-phosphate have been presented. R. R. Brown and co-workers (*Clin. Sci.*, **41**, 237, 1971) did attempt to show a correlation between urinary levels of 4-pyridoxic acid and abnormal excretion of several oxidative metabolites under tryptophan loading.

Kotake and co-workers (*J. Biochem.*, **52**, 162, 1962) were able to show that in rats fed with a vitamin B_6-deficient diet kynurenine transaminase, for the most part in the mitochondria, is inhibited only to 50 per cent, while kynureninase, present only in the soluble protein fraction, loses 75 per cent of its activity. If there is an increased supply of the substrate 3-hydroxykynurenine it is then understandable that xanthurenic acid formation should be increased. However, 3-hydroxyanthranilic acid formation should be lowered at the same time. Furthermore, if it is assumed that the same kynurenine transaminase catalyses the formation of xanthurenic acid and of kynurenic acid, then it is expected that not only xanthurenic acid but also kynurenic acid should be equally formed in increased amounts. The existence of two kynurenine transaminases has not yet been demonstrated.

That is to say, a true vitamin B_6 deficiency should be characterised by reduced amounts of 3-hydroxyanthranilic acid and of anthranilic acid and by proportionally increased amounts of xanthurenic and kynurenic acid.

To return to your direct question: in the case of an acute vitamin B_6 deficiency the metabolites of 3-hydroxyanthranilic acid in the nicotinic acid pathway should be decreased below normal in both the basal and in the urine after a load. As we saw in one of the slides, the values obtained for the metabolites from this pathway, especially those of

N_1-methylnicotinamide and of 2-pyridoneamide, lie entirely within the normal range.

La Du (*New York*). Have you studied the pattern of tryptophan metabolites with or without a load in, say, 10–15 normal individuals to see how uniform the normal group would be?

Byrd. Yes. The control values presented here for the oxidative pathway and for the nicotinic acid pathway were taken from just such a study. The determination of the indole metabolites from the same normal individuals is in progress. Even though the indole study is incomplete I can say that there are also fundamental differences between the controls and the PKUs studied so far.

Perry (*Vancouver*). Dr Byrd, you have divided your patients into two groups; one of which you consider to have classical phenylketonuria and the other 'hyperphenylalaninaemia'. You have arbitrarily taken those patients with plasma phenylalanine below 20 mg/100 ml to have 'hyperphenylalaninaemia'. How do you know that all your patients were not in fact classical phenylketonurics? I note that all were mentally defective. Would it not be wise to check the parents for heterozygosity, by any of the standard tests? Our experience has been with a small group of hyperphenylalaninaemic patients that, using the phenylalanine/tyrosine molar ratio in fasting plasma, one can usually demonstrate that one or both parents are *not* heterozygotes for phenylketonuria, when the patient really has 'hyperphenylalaninaemia'. On the other hand, when the patient has classical phenylketonuria, one should be able to demonstrate that both parents are heterozygotes.

Byrd. The division of our patients into hyperphenylalaninaemics and classical phenylketonurics was not the objective of our study. Our objective was, as I said before, to obtain a general picture of tryptophan metabolism in untreated phenylketonurics. The results of this investigation led to the division of the patients into two groups. The fact that this grouping coincides with the division of the patients into those with serum phenylalanine values of below 20 mg/100 ml and those with values of 20 mg/100 ml and above is an interesting secondary finding. I think that Professor Bickel is in a better position than I am to answer your question on heterozygote tests.

Bickel (*Heidelberg*). Dr Perry, I do not believe that classical phenylketonuria and hyperphenylalaninaemia can usually be differentiated by heterozygote tests on the parents. In PKU these tests are not infallible. More important, we, as well as other authors have found that there are no consistent differences in the heterozygote status of the parents of phenylketonuric as compared to hyperphenylalaninaemic patients.

SCREENING FOR INBORN ERRORS OF METABOLISM USING GAS-LIQUID CHROMATOGRAPHY, MASS SPECTROMETRY AND COMPUTER TECHNIQUE

by

EGIL JELLUM, ODDVAR STOKKE AND LORENTZ ELDJARN

Introduction

ONE of the most powerful analytical tools presently known is the combination of gas-liquid chromatography (GLC) for separation purposes, mass spectrometry (MS) for identification and structure studies, and computer technique (EDP) for data handling. This technique is applicable to all organic compounds which can be made volatile. We have assembled the GLC-MS-EDP methods into a system for multicomponent analysis of urine, serum and other biological materials. The system detects several hundred different metabolites, and can be used to diagnose about 40 presently known inborn errors of metabolism. This systematic screening of about 250 patients, mainly mentally retarded children, has resulted in the discovery of methylmalonic acidaemia (Stokke *et al.*, 1967), and more recently in the discovery of β-hydroxyisovaleric aciduria and β-methylcrotonylglycinuria (Eldjarn *et al.*, 1970), and pyroglutamic aciduria (Jellum *et al.* 1970).

GLC-methods

The detailed description of our instruments, methods of extraction, hydrolysis and derivative formation have been described elsewhere (Jellum, Stokke & Eldjarn, 1971). Only an outline of the analytical procedures, the principles of which are shown in Fig. 1, will therefore be given in the present paper. Urine samples are analysed directly, whereas serum and other biological samples, e.g. biopsies, are first homogenised and treated with ethanol to precipitate the proteins.

Eight different gas chromatograms (A to H) are recorded (Fig. 1). After addition of internal standards, the urine is acidified and extracted with diethyl ether. This extract is used to obtain chromatograms A–D, and further treatment of the aqueous phase yields chromatograms E–H.

All ether-soluble substances that are volatile without derivatisation, such as alcohols, ketones, certain aldehydes, short-chain fatty acids, hydrocarbons etc. are detected on chromatograms A and B. The Porapak P column (system A) is used because it detects the very volatile compounds, e.g. the lower alcohols, acetaldehyde, etc., which on most other GLC columns are eluted together with the solvent front and therefore not

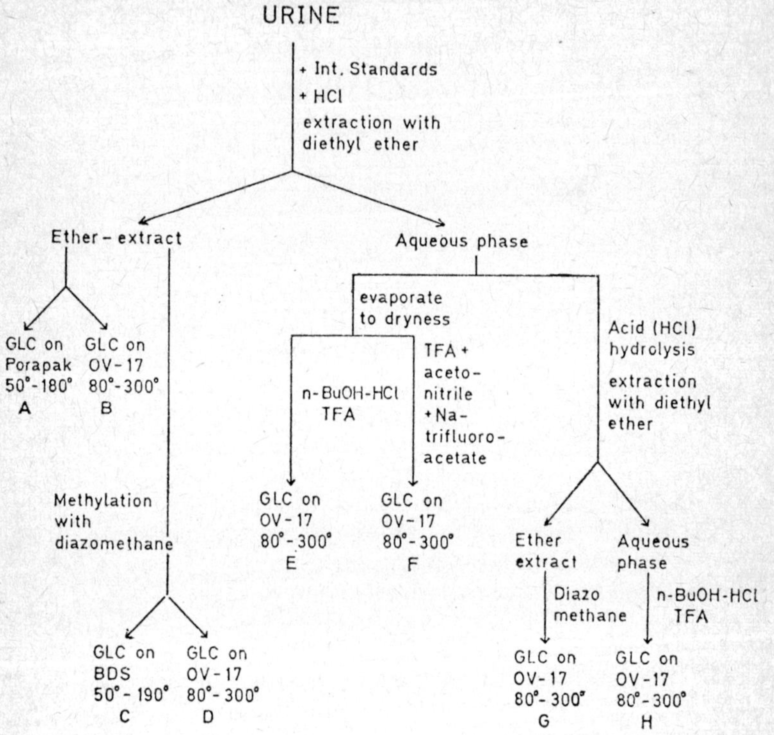

FIG. 1. Principles of the gas-liquid chromatography procedures.

detected. The Porapak column also separates the lower free fatty acids (C_2 to C_8), which are more difficult to analyse on other GLC columns.

The non-derivatised ether extract is also analysed on an OV-17 column (system B). This separates substances which are volatile at higher temperatures, such as higher alcohols, aldehydes, ketones, aliphatic and aromatic hydrocarbons, certain barbiturates and other heterocyclic compounds. The OV-17 column also permits analyses of certain non-esterified fatty acids (C_3 to C_8), although these are better separated on the Porapak column.

GLC systems C and D include a methylation step and detect in general aliphatic as well as aromatic acids (mono-, di-, and tri-carboxylic acids, including the Krebs cycle intermediates). Phenols which are methylated to yield methoxy compounds, are also detected. The methyl derivatives are separated on two columns, a BDS column (system C) and an OV-17 column (system D). These systems, in particular the latter, detect a great number of acidic metabolites. Thus, the chromatographic pattern often shows 50 to 80 peaks in addition to those peaks seen when an unmethylated ether extract is separated on the same column (system B). The BDS column is used because it offers considerably better separation of the saturated and unsaturated higher fatty acids than the less polar OV-17 column.

GLC system E determines amino acids, some simple dipeptides and other ether-insoluble amines. The amino compounds are usually converted into the N-trifluoroacetyl-n-butyl esters before GLC, although sometimes they are also separated as PIV-aldehyde (trimethylacetaldehyde) derivatives (Jellum *et al.*, 1969).

System F detects carbohydrates, including mono-, di- and tri- saccharides, and also certain amino sugars. The carbohydrates are converted into the O-trifluoroacetyl derivatives and separated on an OV-17 column. This method of derivative formation of the sugars is preferred over trimethylsilation, since the latter method would also include the amino acids and thus make the chromatogram unnecessarily complicated.

GLC system G and H include a hydrolysis step. An aliquot of the aqueous phase is refluxed with hydrochloric acid, resulting in hydrolysis of peptides, conjugates and other hydrolysable compounds. The mixture is then extracted with diethyl ether, and both the organic and aqueous phases are used for further analyses. The ether extract is treated with diazomethane, and the methyl esters are separated on an OV-17 column. The resulting chromatogram (system G) detects ether-soluble organic compounds (acids mainly) which have been liberated from conjugates with e.g. glucuronic acid and glycine.

The aqueous phase remaining after ether extraction of the hydrolysed mixture is derivatised with n-butanol/HCl and TFA, and the resulting chromatogram (H) detects the total amino acids, including those liberated by the acid hydrolysis of the urine. Comparison of chromatograms E and H gives information on the amount and amino acid composition of hydrolysable peptides and ether-insoluble amino acid conjugates in the urine.

Mass Spectrometry and Metabolite Identification by Computer Matching

The number of GLC peaks, small and large, on each chromatographic system may be as high as one hundred. With eight GLC systems in operation, it is conceivable that the number of mass spectra per patient may be very large, even if mass spectra are recorded only of the major GLC peaks. Manual interpretation of all the spectra is very difficult and time-consuming, and it was soon realised that a computer had to be included in the system. At the moment we employ an off-line (IBM 1130 computer), and a program has been designed to match unknown mass spectra against a library file of reference spectra, and to print out a list according to the degree of matching. Final verification of the identity of an unknown compound is done by comparison of its complete, original mass spectrum with that of the authentic compound(s) selected by the computer program. At present our library file contains the mass spectra of about 7600 different chemical compounds. New compounds of biological interest are continuously being added to the library, partly by running metabolites through our own GLC-MS system, and partly by selecting MS-spectra from the literature.

Application of the GLC-MS-EDP System on Inborn Errors of Metabolism

The analytical systems described above are now being used extensively in our laboratory for the diagnosis of metabolic errors. The blood and urine samples from the patient suspected of metabolic disease is usually first subjected to a number of standard clinical chemical analyses, such as blood pH, pCO_2, standard bicarbonate, serum and urine urea and uric acid, urinary titratable acid, creatine, creatinine, various stick tests, etc. The sample is then analysed by the GLC-MS-EDP methods. Fresh morning urine or fasting blood samples are always used, in order to minimise diurnal variations and differences in dietary habits. Furthermore, the patient should not have taken any drugs during the week preceding collection of the urine and blood specimens. This is important to avoid abnormal GLC peaks which are due to the drug or its metabolites.

Until now we have used the above scheme to analyse samples from 250-300 patients from different clinical departments of the University Hospitals in Norway, from various Norwegian institutions for mentally retarded children, as well as occasional samples sent to us from hospitals abroad. The system has proved to be a very valuable tool in the diagnosis of known metabolic disorders. This is evident from Table I, which shows that about 40 known inborn errors of metabolism may be diagnosed with the present screening technique. It should be emphasised, however, that proteins, peptides, nucleic acids and their derivatives, porphyrins, bile pigments and a number of other intermediates cannot be analysed by the GLC-MS methods. Thus some inborn errors of protein metabolism, of red-cell metabolism, of pigment and mineral metabolism will consequently escape detection in the present system.

The GLC-MS-EDP system is also a most valuable tool for the detailed study of the abnormal metabolism in patients with an inborn error. Thus we have extensively used gas chromatography and mass spectrometry technique to pinpoint the enzymatic defect in Refsum's disease (Stokke, Try & Eldjarn, 1967), and to study the defect in congenital lactic acidosis (Skrede *et al.*, 1971).

The system has proved potent in the discovery of new inborn errors of metabolism, i.e. those resulting in accumulation or excretion of metabolites which are volatile, or can be converted into volatile derivatives. Examples of this application is the discovery of methylmalonic acidaemia,

Table I. *Inborn errors of metabolism detectable by the screening system*

Name of disease	*Compounds detectable by the GLC-MS methods*
Alcaptonuria	homogentisic acid
Carnosinaemia	carnosine
Congenital lactacidosis	lactic acid
Cystathioninuria	cystathionine
Cystinuria	cystine
Diabetes mellitus	glucose, β-hydroxybutyric acid, acetoacetic acid
Essential fructosuria	fructose
Essential pentosuria	L-xylulose
Galactosaemia	galactose, amino acids
L-glyceric aciduria	L-glyceric acid, oxalic acid
Hartnup disease	neutral amino acids
Histidinaemia	histidine, imidazoleacetic acid
Homocystinuria	homocystine, methionine
β-Hydroxyisovaleric aciduria & β- methylcrotonylglycinuria	β-hydroxyisovaleric acid, β-methylcrotonylglycine
Hydroxylysinuria	hydroxylysine
Hydroxyprolinaemia	hydroxyproline
Hyper-β-alaninaemia	β-alanine, β-aminoisobutyric acid, δ-aminobutyric acid
Hyperlysinaemia	lysine
Hypermethioninaemia	methionine, α-keto-δ-methiolbutyric acid
Hyperoxaluria	oxalic acid, glycolic acid, glyoxylic acid
Hyperprolinaemia	proline
Hypersarcosinaemia	sarcosine
Hypertryptophanaemia	tryptophane
Hypervalinaemia	valine
Isovaleric acidaemia	isovaleric acid, β-hydroxyisovaleric acid, isovalerylglycine
Maple syrup urine disease	valine, leucine, isoleucine, α-ketoisovaleric acid, α-ketoisocaproic acid, α-keto-β-methylvaleric acid
Methylmalonic acidaemia	methylmalonic acid
Non-ketotic hyperglycinaemia	glycine
Oast-House disease	α-hydroxybutyric acid
Ornithinaemia	ornithine
Orotic aciduria	orotic acid
Phenylketonuria	phenylalanine, phenylpyruvic acid, phenyllactic acid, o-hydroxyphenyl-acetic acid
Propionic acidaemia	propionic acid
Pyroglutamic aciduria	pyroglutamic acid (pyrrolidone-2-carboxylic acid)
Refsum's disease	phytanic acid
Renal glycosuria	glucose
Short chain fatty acidaemia	butyric acid, caproic acid
Tyrosinosis	tyrosine, p-hydroxyphenylpyruvic acid, p-hydroxyphenyllactic acid

which we (Stokke *et al.*, 1967) made simultaneously and independently of Oberholzer *et al.* (1967). More recently we have discovered β-hydroxyisovaleric aciduria and β-methylcrotonylglycinuria (Eldjarn *et al.*, 1970, see also paper by Stokke, Jellum & Eldjarn in this symposium) and pyroglutamic aciduria (Jellum *et al.*, 1970, see also paper by Eldjarn, Stokke & Jellum in this symposium).

Conclusion

The GLC-MS-EDP technique is at present rapidly expanding into hospitals and clinical chemistry. This methodology will undoubtedly result in a better understanding of a number of metabolic errors, and will probably also result in the discovery of further inborn errors of metabolism as well as genetic variants. It should be borne in mind, however, that the system is limited to metabolites which can be made volatile. Other methods, such as high-speed liquid chromatography, must therefore be used for analyses of non-volatile compounds.

REFERENCES

Eldjarn, L., Jellum, E., Stokke, O., Pande, H. & Waaler, P. E. (1970) *Lancet*, **ii**, 521.
Jellum, E., Close, V. A., Patton, W., Pereira, W. & Halpern, B. (1969) *Anal. Biochem.*, **31**, 227.
Jellum, E., Kluge, T., Børresen, H. C. Stokke, O & Eldjarn, L. (1970) *Scand. J. clin. Lab. Invest.*, **26**, 327.
Jellum, E., Stokke, O. & Eldjarn, L. (1971) *Scand. J. clin. Lab. Invest.*, **27**, 273.
Oberholzer, B., Levin, E., Burgess, A. & Young, W. (1967) *Arch. Dis. Childh.*, **42**, 492.
Skrede, S., Strömme, J. H., Stokke, O., Lie, S. O. & Eldjarn, L. (1971) *Acta paediat. Scand.*, **60**, 138.
Stokke, O., Eldjarn, L., Norum, K. R., Steen-johnson, J. & Halvorsen, S. (1967) *Scand. J. clin. Lab. Invest.*, **20**, 313.
Stokke, O., Try, K. & Eldjarn, L. (1967) *Biochim. biophys, Acta*, **144**, 271.

DISCUSSION
(of the Paper by Dr Jellum)

Watts (*Harrow*). The initial fractionation by partition between the organic solvent ether and water is inevitably inefficient from the point of view of extraction of the very hydrophilic compounds which may be of great interest in the study of inborn errors of metabolism. How do you overcome this?

How do you handle the link between the gas chromatograph and mass spectrometer, what type of mass spectrometer do you use, what is its maximum resolution, and what resolution do you use routinely?

To what extent do you depend on absolute mass measurement for identification, can you sample different regions of a single GLC peak?

Your slide listed forty-one disorders which may be diagnosed by your technique. How many inborn errors have, in fact, been identified by your system?

Jellum (*Oslo*). It is of course true that many compounds, for instance hydroxy acids and di- and tri-carboxylic acid are poorly extracted by diethyl ether. It is evident from the scheme shown in the slide, however, that we always analyse both the organic and the aqueous phase. Incompletely extractable compounds are therefore detected in two of the GLC systems. May I add that we now have started experiments where extractions are being replaced by anion and cation exchange clean-up procedures.

The equipment we use comprises a Varian CH 7 mass spectrometer, to which a Varian 1400 gas chromatograph is connected via a molecular separator of the glass-frit type. The resolution we use routinely is about 1:1200, although it can be increased to 1:3000 by changing slits. The instrument is quite capable of recording mass spectra at different regions of a single GLC peak to establish its homogeneity.

In cases where the mass spectrum of an unknown GLC peak is not recognised by the computer and is not listed in any of mass spectral data collections, we usually carry out 'manual' interpretation of the low resolution mass spectrum. If this also is a failure, we fortunately have access to a high resolution mass spectrometer at the Chemistry Department of Oslo University. It is quite clear that a high resolution instrument, which gives absolute masses and empirical formulæ, at the present stage is of great help in detection of new metabolic errors. However, I believe that when more and more biochemical and clinical chemistry laboratories begin to use GLC-MS-computer methods, the collection of known mass spectra will increase vastly, so that practically every described metabolite and biochemical compound (which are volatile) will be recognised by the computer. When this stage is reached, the need for a high resolution instrument will decrease.

With regard to your last question, I must admit that we have only come across and diagnosed about fifteen of the forty-one metabolic errors listed in the slide. However, all the pathological metabolites shown in the table are indeed detectable by our systems.

Cusworth (*London*). This apparatus is very expensive for screening. How many of the forty or so disorders which you can detect in this way can also be detected with a test tube and a piece of blotting paper?

Jellum. The advantage of using GLC-MS for the diagnosis of the forty inborn errors listed in the table, is that one single set of analyses is capable of detecting any one of these disorders. To my knowledge this cannot be done with a test tube and a piece of blotting paper. In Scandinavia, at least, we would probably have to use forty test tubes, forty blotting papers and forty different methods to obtain the same result.

I would like to emphasise that our analytical set-up by no means are primarily meant to be used for screening and diagnosis of well-known metabolic errors. It is the detection of new and unknown disorders that are especially facilitated by the GLC-MS-computer methods. I am quite sure that for instance the identification of β-methylcrotonylglycine, which has not been detected in biological materials before, would be rather difficult with the help of a test tube and a blotting paper.

I would also like to point out that we consider the application of GLC-MS-computer method to inborn errors as merely one aspect of its uses. To our mind it is quite clear that such a technique is going to play a more and more important role in clinical chemistry in general. We believe that detailed information on the metabolic patterns of patients may give valuable information on many diseases. I may therefore add that apart from inborn errors, we are at the moment working on projects using GLC-MS-computer methods in cancer research, in studies on ketosis, and in studies on hepatic disorders.

Gompertz (*London*). There is a place for techniques of complexity between that of paper chromatography and sophisticated GLC mass spectrometry. I have in mind the use of ordinary gas chromatographs at low amplification to screen for 'abnormal peaks'. Once a peak has been found GLC mass spectrometry is essential. However, a lot of useful screening can be performed with simple gas chromatography.

CHROMATOGRAPHIC SCREENING METHODS FOR ORGANIC ACIDS IN URINE

by

J. W. T. SEAKINS

Introduction

The clinical chemist is faced with a somewhat difficult task in providing methods for the detection of inborn errors of metabolism (other than PKU). Not only is the incidence of the various diseases very low, even in a population of hospitalised children, but spot tests which might eliminate normal results are either not reliable (e.g. ferric chloride) or not available. It is hardly surprising that complicated methods have been suggested for the screening of a wide variety of substances in one single procedure. For example, Scott and his collaborators (e.g. Jolley & Scott, 1970) have described column methods for separating UV absorbing substances in urine, which employ pressures of up to 4000 lb/in^2 (280 kg/cm^2) and take 24 hours for each run. Likewise Dalgliesh and co-workers (1966) originally devised their gas-liquid chromatographic separations to detect a wide range of solvent-extractable substances present in urine.

Good though these methods may be, they demand expensive equipment, and are limited in the number of samples that can be processed. Our approach has been rather to apply several simple chromatographic methods as a preliminary screening, and then to apply more sophisticated methods to the abnormal specimens. In this paper, some aspects of the methods we have employed are discussed, and also the contribution of dietary substances, 'anutrients', to the aromatic acid chromatogram. The final section summarises some recent work on the origin of phenylacetyl glutamine.

It is assumed that PKU, homocystinuria (methionine) and possibly histidinaemia have been eliminated by suitable screening methods, for example Guthrie's inhibition assay or its chromatographic equivalent, and that plasma and urinary amino acid patterns have been determined. Ready-prepared thin layers of silica-gel and *crystalline* cellulose on flexible foils are now commercially available. The greater resolution and increased sensitivity afforded by these layers have facilitated these studies, by reducing or eliminating sample preparation, and shortening running time. Abnormalities in these patterns will obviously suggest further investigations, for example an elevated plasma tyrosine would indicate urinary phenolic and keto acids, a raised plasma glycine would suggest tests for methylmalonic and propionic acids.

Aromatic Acids

It was found that simple ether extraction of the acidified urine sample which had been saturated with ammonium sulphate was adequate for two-way thin layer chromatography of phenolic acids (Ersser *et al.*, 1970). Fig. 1 demonstrates that there is no loss in resolving power when 5 cm squares are used. Fig. 2 illustrates some typical separations. The time taken for complete operation, including preparing the sample is about 2 hours and the cost (excluding labour) 2 new pence. The corresponding paper method (25 cm square sheets) takes about 36 hours and gives inferior resolution. (The ether extract may be used to screen for methylmalonic acid by the method of Gutteridge and Wright, 1970; adequate separation is obtained in a 4 cm run.)

In the literature on the GLC of urinary aromatic acids various solvents have been advocated for extraction of urine. Again, we have found ether extraction of acidified urine which has been saturated with ammonium sulphate brings out all the important aromatic metabolites that can be directly separated by GLC, and leaves in the aqueous layer substances such as phenylacetyl glutamine (see below), urea, glucuronides, pigments which can interfere with subsequent trimethylsillation. However, simple ether or ethyl acetate extraction may be inadequate for isolating non-volatile aliphatic acids, particularly the acyl glycines. Thus propionyl glycine can be recrystallised from ethyl acetate.

Since diazomethane is a hazardous toxic substance which can give rise to aromatic methyl ethers as well as the desired methyl ester, we have employed trimethylsilyl ether/ester derivatives. On the whole, these derivatives are well separated on columns of OV-1 and OV-17, and the difference in polarity of the two phases is an aid to identification (Coward & Smith, 1969). Nevertheless, the separation and quantitation of important metabolites may be difficult; for example, on OV-17 phenyllactic and o-hydroxyphenylacetic acids run together, but separate from m-hydroxybenzoic acid. p-hydroxyphenylacetic acid is separated from p-hydroxybenzoic acid on OV-17, but inadequately on OV-1. Vanillic and homovanillic acids and their isomers are poorly separated from each other on either column. For 4-hydroxy-3-methoxymandelic acid (VMA) it may be necessary to oxidise the VMA to vanillin which can then be determined by GLC to obtain the necessary specificity (compare Van de Calseyde *et al.*, 1971).

Dietary Sources of Urinary Organic Acids

In normal persons, vegetables, fruits and beverages are by far the major sources of urinary phenolic acids, and possibly some aliphatic acids. These sources contain a wide range of aromatic compounds; simple phenolic acids and esters and aldehydes, flavonoid compounds, tannins

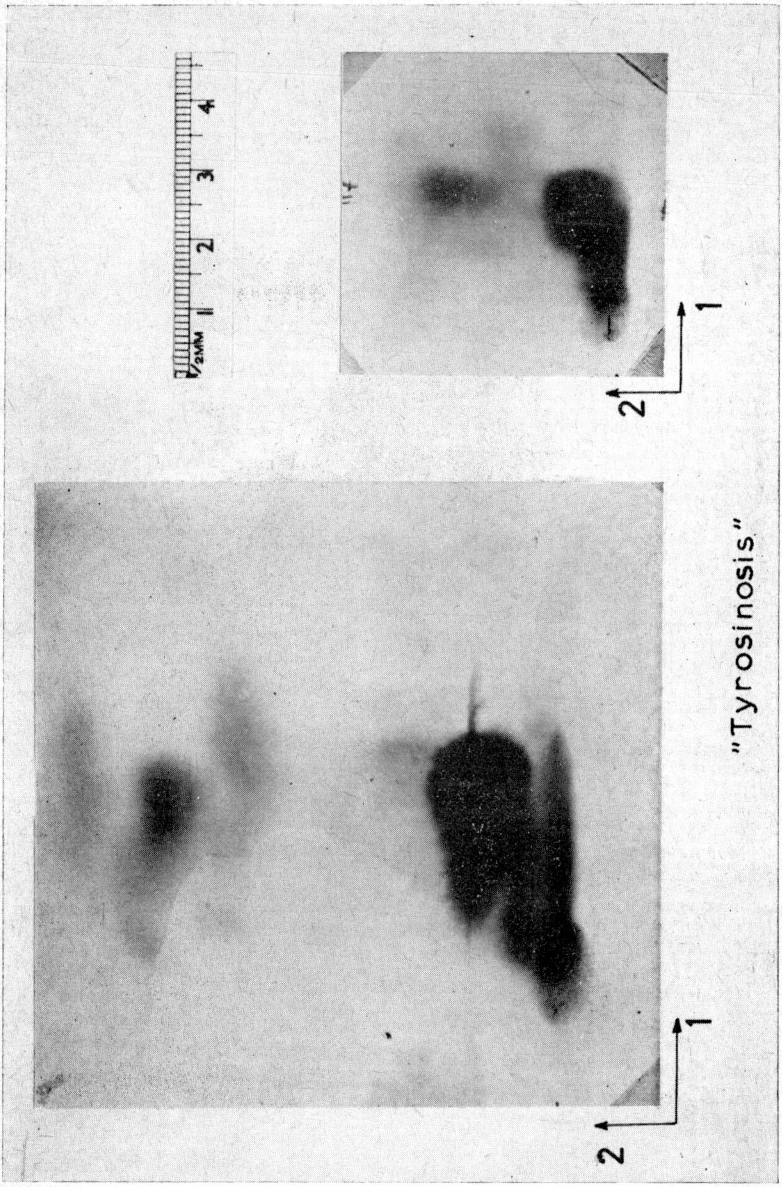

FIG. 1. Urinary phenolic acids: Comparison of the same pathological urine extract on 10 cm and 5 cm squares. Chromatogram sprayed with diazotised sulphanilic acid.

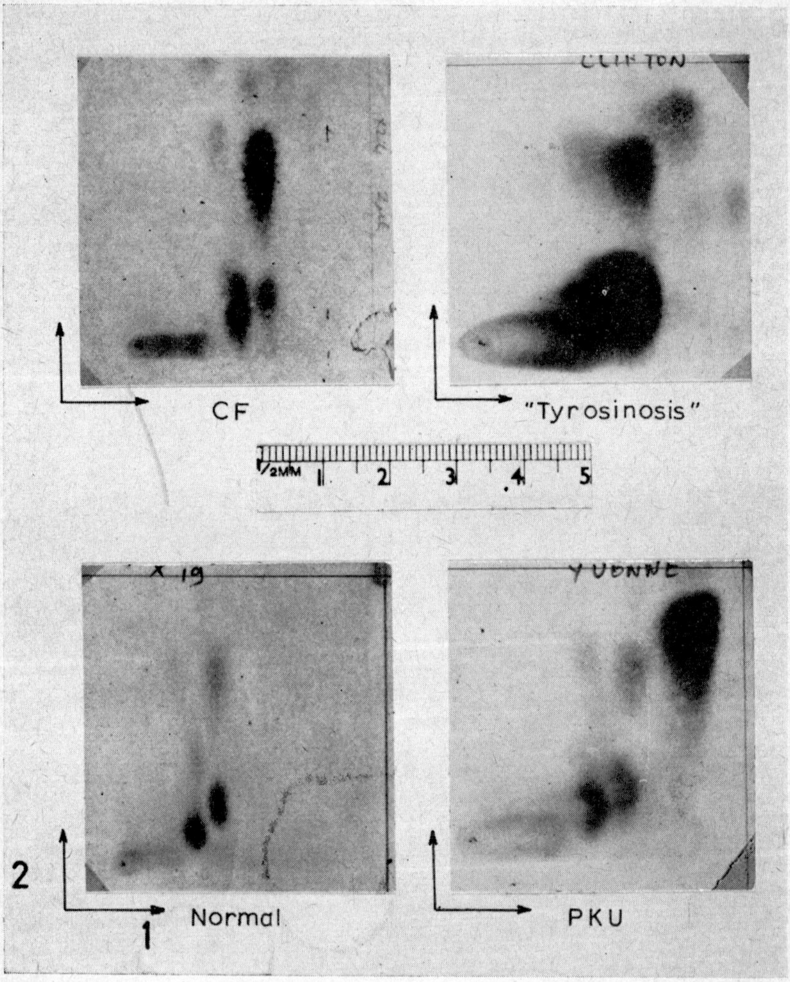

FIG. 2. *Solvent 1*: Isopropanol-n-butanol-t-butanol-ammonia (0·88) water (40:20:20:10:20) 22 minutes.
Solvent 2: Benzene-acetic acid-water (70:29:1) 6 minutes.
Normal subject: m-hydroxyhippuric and m-hydroxyhydacrylic acids.
Cystic fibrosis: *p*-hydroxyphenylacetic acid (dominant).
Phenylketonuria; o-hydroxyphenylacetic acid.
Tyrosinosis: *p*-hydroxyphenyllactic acid with lesser amounts of *p*-hydroxymandelic and *p*-hydroxyphenylacetic acids.

and lignins; and also aliphatic compounds which can be converted into aromatic acids. Orange juice (Kefford & Chandler, 1970) and blackcurrant juice (Morton, 1968) are particularly rich in these substances and are consumed in vast quantities as sources of vitamin C or given to mask unpleasant flavours, etc.

Simple phenolic compounds are absorbed direct from the stomach and/or small intestine, and may be excreted unchanged, conjugated with glycine, glucuronide or sulphate, or undergo methylation, etc. More complex substances such as the flavonoids and their glycosides, quinic acid esters are poorly absorbed from the small bowel, and are degraded in the large bowel to simpler phenolic substances, where in addition demethylation and p-dehydroxylation can also occur, and quinic acid is converted to benzoic acid (Adamson *et al.*, 1970). Benzoic acid may, under some circumstances, be a gut metabolite of phenylalanine (Van der Heiden *et al.*, 1971).

Fig. 3, which summarises the metabolism of chlorogenic acid, a major phenolic constituent of coffee, illustrates some of these alternative pathways. Dayman and Jepson (1969) found that ingested caffeic acid resulted in the rapid excretion of o-methylated phenolic acids, whereas the excretion of m-hydroxy acids was delayed many hours. Other examples are given in Smith *et al.* (1969).

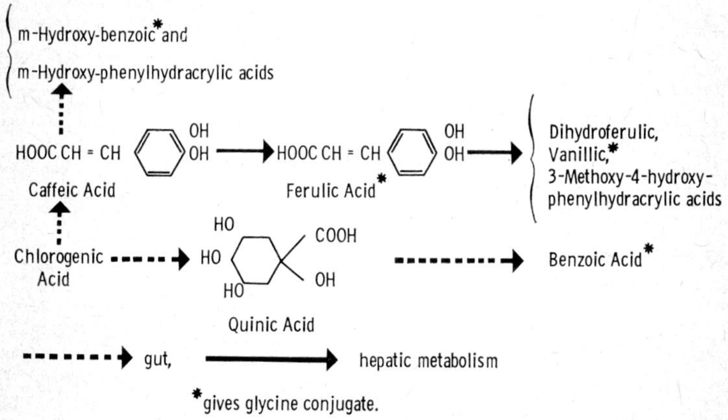

FIG. 3. The metabolism of chlorogenic acid.

Complicated phenolic compounds such as the flavonoids which have been absorbed intact are probably excreted as glucuronides (cf. Williams, 1959), and as such may be extracted from urine and interfere with subsequent chromatographic procedures. The determination of the basal excretion of important metabolites can thus be made difficult in the absence of strict dietary control. For example, the flavonone glycoside hesperedin present in citrus fruits gives rise to isovanilloyl glycine and isovanilloyl hydacrylic acid, both of which interfere with the paper chromatographic determination of VMA (Smith, 1962). Orange juice can also give rise to metabolites with paper chromatographic properties and colour reactions similar to but not identical with p-hydroxyphenyl-acetic and -lactic acids (Seakins, unpublished). Quercetin and its glycosides, e.g. rutin, are present in blackcurrants and apples and are degraded to homovanillic and m-hydroxyphenyl acetic acids (Williams, 1959).

Origin of Phenylacetyl Glutamine

Phenylacetylglutamine (PAG) is an important aromatic metabolite and accounts for about half the bound glutamine (or glutamic acid) in human urine (Stein *et al.*, 1954). It was nearly 60 years ago in Germany that Sherwin began his extensive studies on the metabolism of phenylacetic acid and related compounds, which he was to continue with many colleagues over the next twenty years in U.S.A. (summarised by Williams, 1959). They showed that PAG was the major metabolite of ingested phenylacetic acid and β-phenylethylamine in humans. Power and Sherwin (1927) further suggested that urinary PAG was a putrefactive end product of phenylalanine metabolism (Fig. 4,A). In contrast, Woolf (1963) following the observation of Stein *et al.* (1954) that the excretion of PAG did not alter during (? a short) fast, stated that urinary PAG in the normal subject was an endogenous end-product of phenylalanine metabolism, formed as in PKU, via phenylpyruvic acid (Fig. 4, B).

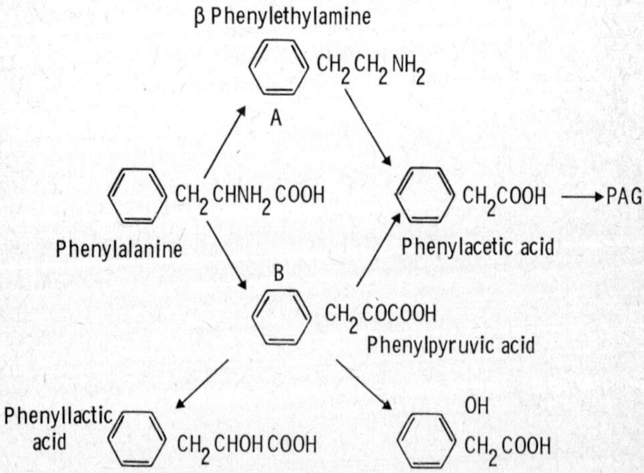

FIG. 4. Formation of phenylacetylglutamine.

Investigations into the origin of PAG have been hampered by lack of suitable methods for its determination. Gas-chromatographic determination of phenylacetic acid liberated by alkaline hydrolysis has provided a rapid and convenient method (Seakins, 1971). Independently, similar hydrolysis methods have been published by Van der Heiden *et al.* (1971); and Vavich and Howell (1971).

Our results can be summarised as follows (Seakins, 1971). If PAG is an end-product of endogenous phenylalanine metabolism, then, by analogy with phenylketonuria (Woolf, 1963) significant quantities of phenyllactic and -pyruvic acids should be found in normal urine. However, GLC failed to detect either metabolite; and even during a load of D-phenylalanine, when there was considerable output of phenylpyruvic acid, the excretion of PAG was only slightly increased. As found by Power and Sherwin, ingested phenylacetic acid and β-phenylethylamine were rapidly and quantitatively excreted as PAG, but a load of L-phenylalanine gave an even smaller rise in PAG than did D-phenylalanine. These observations indicated that either PAG arose from exogenous phenylalanine metabolism, or there were dietary non-protein sources. The latter were excluded and when an enzymic hydrolysate of lactalbumin was substituted as the sole source of protein, the excretion of PAG fell to a quarter of the base line value, 30 hours after the institution of the dietary change, and 40 hours after the last normal meal. Young (1970) has observed a fall in the excretion of PAG to one-fifth base-line values following the institution of a purely synthetic diet. The suggestion of Power and Sherwin (1927) over 40 years ago that PAG in the normal subject is a 'putrefactive' end-product of phenylalanine metabolism has thus been confirmed, and the phenylalanine is derived from unabsorbed protein residues mostly dietary in origin. Although Moldave and Meister (1957) found that human liver homogenates converted phenylalanine into PAG in the presence of appropriate substrates, the results from the phenylalanine loads rule out this pathway in the normal human subject.

Since PAG is derived ultimately from gut metabolism, its excretion might be elevated in patients where protein malabsorption is not associated with excessive intestinal hurry as exemplified by cystic fibrosis (Seakins *et al.*, 1970), thus allowing bacterial proteolysis and decarboxylation, etc., to take place freely. This was found to be so in about half the urine specimens from twelve children with cystic fibrosis. Van Der Heiden *et al.* (1971) also reported gross excretion of PAG in one patient with cystic fibrosis who had severe malabsorption, and of particular interest was the finding of phenylacetic acid in the faeces.

Acknowledgements

The author wishes to thank the Cystic Fibrosis Research Foundation Trust for financial assistance and Mr R. S. Ersser, F.I.M.L.T., for valuable discussion.

REFERENCES

ADAMSON, R. H., BRIDGES, J. W., EVANS, M. E. & WILLIAMS, R. T. (1970) *Biochem. J.*, **116**, 437.

COWARD, R. F. & SMITH, P. (1969) *J. Chromatogr.*, **45**, 230.

DALGLIESH, C. E., HORNING, E. C., HORNING, M. G., KNOX, K. L. & YARGER, K. (1966) *Biochem. J.*, **101**, 792.
DAYMAN, J. & JEPSON, J . B. (1969) *Biochem. J.*, **113**, 11.
ERSSER, R. S., OAKLEY, S. E. & SEAKINS, J. W. T. (1970) *Clin. chim. Acta*, **30**, 243.
GUTTERIDGE, J. M. & WRIGHT, E. B. (1970) *Clin. chim. Acta*, **27**, 289.
JOLLEY, R. L. & SCOTT, C. D. (1970) *Clin. Chem.*, **16**, 687.
KEFFORD, J. F. & CHANDLER, B. V. (1970) *The Chemical Constituents of Citrus Fruits*. New York: Academic Press.
MOLDAVE, K. & MEISTER, A. (1957) *J. biol. Chem.*, **229**, 463.
MORTON, A. D. (1968) *J. Fd Technol.*, **3**, 269.
Power, F. W. & SHERWIN, C. P. (1927) *Arch. int. Med.*, **39**, 60.
SEAKINS, J. W. T. (1971) *Clin. chim. Acta*, in the press.
SEAKINS, J. W. T., ERSSER, R. S. & GIBBONS, I. S. E. (1970) *Gut*, **11**, 600.
SMITH, I., SEAKINS, J. W. T. & DAYMAN, J. (1969) *In* Smith, I. *Chromatographic and Electrophoretic Techniques*, Vol. 1, London: Heinemann, ch. 16.
SMITH, P. (1962) *In* Varley H. & Gowenlock, A. H., *Clinical Chemistry of Monoamines*. Amsterdam: Elsevier, p. 31.
STEIN, W. H., PALADINI, A. C., HIRS, C. H. W. & MOORE, S. (1954) *J. amer. chem. Soc.*, **76**, 2848.
VAN DE CALSEYDE, J. P., SCHOLTIS, R. J. H., SCHMIDT, N. A. & LEYTON, C. J. J. A. (1971) *Clin. chim. Acta*, **32**, 361.
VAN DER HEIDEN, C., WADMAN, S. K., KETTING. D. & DE BREE, P. K. (1971) *Clin. chim. Acta*, **31**, 133.
VAVICH, J. M. & HOWELL, R. R. (1971) *J. Lab. clin. Med.*, **77**, 159.
WILLIAMS, R. T. (1959) *Detoxication Mechanisms*, 2nd ed. London: Chapman & Hall.
WOOLF, L. I. (1963) *Advanc: clin. Chem.*, **6**, 97 Inherited metabolic disorders: errors of phenylalanine and tyrosine metabolism. *In Advances in Clinical Chemistry*, **6**, New York: Academic Press, 106.
YOUNG, D. S. (1970) *Clin. Chem.*, **16**, 681.

DISCUSSION
(of the Paper by Dr Seakins)

Curtius (*Zurich*). How soon after the consumption of coffee do metabolites appear in the urine?

Seakins (*London*). Some of the phenolic constituents of coffee are readily absorbed from the stomach and small intestine, and rapidly metabolized and excreted. The main phenolic constituent chlorogenic acid, the caffeic acid ester of quinic acid, is poorly absorbed. In the large bowel it undergoes hydrolysis and the liberated caffeic acid is either absorbed as such or undergoes further bacterial transformations prior to absorption; quinic acid is converted to benzoic acid and absorbed. The excretion of metabolites released or formed in the large bowel takes place approximately 6–24 hours after ingestion. The early morning specimen may therefore be relatively rich in metabolites derived from bacterial transformations in the gut.

Jellum (*Oslo*). I agree that diet is very important. A standard diet would be ideal for our purposes but this is not practicable. We therefore use fresh morning specimens of urine, which are relatively characteristic of the endogenous metabolism.